Sterile Processing

Word Puzzles

Volume 1 **Leadership & Culture**

Beyond Clean

Hank Balch

wenpublishing.com

Word Puzzles created by Janet Bristeir WEN Publishing ©

Sterile Processing Word Puzzles Vol.1 Leadership & Culture

ISBB: 978-1-990599-00-2

Praise for Beyond Clean Podcast

I love the knowledge this crew has and is making publicly available. Using the resources, they are linking together we have had more success in arguing for change in our system. Kevin R.

This is a great resource for SPD professionals, influencers, and educators. Susie C.

Beyond Clean is a vital tool for any Sterile Processing Technician! They hold a wealth of knowledge that can be used by the newest of the new or the ones who've been around the block. Ken B.

Beyond Clean is a must listen! [They] bring the listener into the world of reprocessing – providing an insiders look that is perfect for both the layperson and professional alike. I can't recommend Beyond Clean enough! Do yourself a favor and subscribe! Sarah E.

Introduction

Why create a book of Sterile Processing word puzzles and articles? We asked ourselves a similar question in the summer of 2017, but at that time the question was, "Why launch a podcast about all things Sterile Processing?" Our answer to both of these questions is the same: to *educate*, *engage*, and *innovate* within the medical device reprocessing industry. By the fall of 2021, our weekly podcast had been downloaded over 600,000 times in more than 150 countries around the globe, so it appears we made the right decision. This book project has the potential to make a unique industry impact all its own. With 52 word puzzles developed from 26 of our revolutionary Beyond Clean podcast episodes, this work provides a fun, engaging opportunity to think through the key concepts from each episode and learn a thing or two along the way. The best part? Each puzzle is linked to the actual podcast audio through a custom QR code, allowing you to scan the code and pull up the interview while you work through the puzzle.

In true Beyond Clean style, we took this book one step beyond just a great word puzzle book. Scattered throughout these pages you will find additional articles highlighting important themes in department leadership, recruiting, and culture that were written to help you prepare for career growth and opportunity as a Sterile Processing professional, at whatever stage you find yourself in today.

Finally, we got these articles approved for five (5) continuing education credits for both HPSA (Healthcare Sterile Processing Association) & CBSPD (Certification Board for Sterile Processing & Distribution) certification holders. So, once you finish reading each article, you can visit the link below to take a quick comprehension quiz and print out your CE certificate. https://www.flexiquiz.com/SC/N/volume1

On behalf of our entire team at Beyond Clean, and the millions of patients around the globe who are impacted by the work of Sterile Processing technicians and vendors, I would like to thank you for all you do to #FightDirty, every instrument, every time. I hope you enjoy this book and I look forward to more to come!

Industry Certifications, Research Studies on Certification Impact, The Power of Data

https://directory.libsyn.com/episode/index/id/5789908

Industry Certifications, Research Studies

The Power of Data

Z	S	C	Q	W	U	D	S	A	Q	E	U	C	R	E	X
R	A	I	R	F	E	D	U	C	A	T	I	O	N	P	Z
E	X	P	K	E	R	S	U	N	P	Q	J	A	R	Z	T
J	J	H	D	L	D	W	Z	L	P	N	I	A	T	H	O
S	Z	A	Q	G	A	E	E	W	Z	P	C	Y	C	W	T
C	B	F	M	V	Z	A	N	V	G	T	B	R	H	S	C
I	B	Q	C	A	R	F	J	T	I	G	A	E	Z	A	J
T	Z	O	L	N	X	P	Q	C	I	E	M	G	G	R	U
S	U	Y	I	Y	E	E	E	A	S	A	J	R	O	D	D
I	T	N	N	R	U	A	U	E	T	U	L	U	B	D	E
T	G	T	I	D	L	O	R	T	G	A	F	S	L	R	U
A	C	S	C	R	A	O	V	K	S	L	D	P	Y	I	Q
T	N	A	A	R	V	K	N	O	I	T	C	E	F	N	I
S	N	W	L	P	C	O	M	P	E	T	E	N	C	Y	O
J	A	U	U	G	N	I	S	R	U	N	P	P	I	Q	K
V	N	O	I	T	A	C	I	F	I	T	R	E	C	V	F

CERTIFICATION
CREDENTIAL
COMPETENCY
VALUE
RESEARCH
PRACTICE
NURSING
INFECTION
SURGERY
LEARNING
EXAM
CLINICAL
DATA
EDUCATION
STATISTICS

The Power of Data

Industry Certifications, Research Studies on Certification Impact

CRAIETCOFITIN
4 20

PCRIACTE
8 19

AEMX
21

CERNATEDIL
5

NRNIUSG

CINICALL
11

CPENEOCMTY
18 22

IFIOENCTN
2 16 13

AADT

UVELA

SGERURY
17 6

ECAITOUDN
12

RECASERH
9

LNRIENAG

STISITACTS
23 3 10 14

B																					
1	2	3	4	5	6	8	9	10	11	12	13	14	16	17	18	19	20	21	22	23	

The CS Professional as a Patient, Lessons in Leadership, and Surgical Instrument Quality

https://directory.libsyn.com/episode/index/id/5843190

The CS Professional as a Patient

Lessons in Leadership and Surgical Instrument Quality

C	F	U	F	O	L	P	E	W	J	U	Q	B	B	V	P
T	W	L	P	C	C	C	J	V	Q	N	B	D	B	T	U
R	Q	N	S	L	O	U	E	R	A	C	E	Y	Q	S	P
Z	S	V	O	N	E	R	L	D	N	V	Z	K	S	Y	K
T	I	W	O	E	O	S	V	T	E	W	F	X	F	T	F
T	T	W	B	T	G	O	S	L	U	M	Y	M	Y	T	L
W	S	I	N	M	C	R	O	O	O	R	S	N	T	R	A
Z	S	E	N	A	H	P	U	C	N	R	E	E	I	U	N
Z	M	E	T	F	M	O	L	S	O	S	X	T	L	S	O
R	B	E	N	E	E	E	Y	D	P	A	P	K	A	T	I
J	K	Q	N	Z	A	C	N	E	M	A	H	T	U	L	T
S	O	T	P	R	K	E	T	P	T	C	W	A	Q	G	A
O	X	P	N	S	V	G	L	I	W	G	Y	K	M	B	U
Z	D	G	B	C	T	E	E	K	O	H	N	J	Z	N	T
V	Q	O	C	I	B	N	L	A	E	N	A	F	M	D	I
A	Y	Y	D	Z	T	M	F	V	V	H	T	I	A	Z	S

PATIENT
QUALITY
VENDORS
LEARN
CARE

TRUST
SURGEON
LESSONS
MENTOR
EXAMPLE

CULTURE
INFECTION
SITUATIONAL
DEVELOPMENT
ADVOCATE

The CS Professional as a Patient

Lessons in Leadership and Surgical Instrument Quality

Scrambled word	Numbered boxes
PINETAT	21, 14, 20
UTTRS	3
CRULUTE	
QTIAULY	
SEGUORN	7, 16
IINCTFOEN	9
VNDREOS	6
LSOSNES	12, 18, 5, 10, 4
ANREL	17
MNTOER	
DLPEMVNEOET	15, 13, 1
EPMXLAE	2
AOTVDCAE	

1	2	3	4	5	6	7		9	10		12	13	14	15	16	17	18	19	20	21
																		H		

Business Training for SPD Leaders & Thermal Validation

https://directory.libsyn.com/episode/index/id/6172310

Business Training for SPD Leaders

Thermal Validation

S	R	H	E	G	L	N	O	I	T	A	D	I	L	A	V
R	A	D	M	I	N	I	S	T	R	A	T	I	O	N	S
T	E	A	Y	H	P	I	K	V	P	X	P	U	A	W	Q
N	S	G	S	T	N	E	M	U	R	T	S	N	I	U	V
R	T	O	A	N	R	F	H	R	X	T	S	A	A	G	G
T	E	I	W	N	D	O	E	D	B	T	T	L	X	P	W
O	R	N	Q	D	A	P	Z	W	E	A	I	K	D	R	J
O	I	D	I	P	O	M	L	A	D	F	M	C	N	O	A
G	L	I	Z	R	I	O	M	L	I	M	B	I	A	C	T
V	I	C	T	O	I	S	X	C	O	T	L	J	C	E	C
R	Z	A	Z	Y	H	Y	A	N	M	C	G	C	L	S	U
W	E	T	Q	J	X	T	E	W	V	J	P	B	D	S	D
E	R	O	D	V	I	Y	U	H	G	Q	Z	I	M	I	O
Y	F	R	O	O	S	P	V	D	O	Y	H	D	G	N	R
B	R	B	N	S	S	E	N	I	S	U	B	U	P	G	P
T	H	O	S	P	I	T	A	L	F	C	P	Q	W	R	X

MANAGER
STERILIZER
PROCESSING
DATA
REPORT

MONEY
STEAM
HOSPITAL
INDICATOR
ADMINISTRATION

PRODUCT
INSTRUMENTS
VALIDATION
BUSINESS
QUALIFICATION

Business Training for SPD Leaders

Thermal Validation

MAEGNAR (1, 3, 5)

YEMNO (14)

POCRDUT (20)

SIIETRZLER (6)

ESMTA (13)

ITRNUNTSMES (17, 7)

PISRSCONEG (11, 8)

HIPTSAOL (19)

VLADITOAIN (2)

ATDA (21, 4)

IINCTDOAR (16)

BESUSNIS

RREPOT

AMNOITITASRIDN (10, 12)

QFUICIOTLAIAN

1 2 3 4 5 6 7 8   10 11 12 13 14   16 17   19 20 21

OR/SPD Collaboration & The OR Today Live Conference

https://directory.libsyn.com/episode/index/id/6198160

OR/SPD Collaboration

The OR Today Live Conference

E	T	R	A	N	S	P	A	R	E	N	C	Y	C	O	F
E	D	L	G	Z	T	P	P	W	M	S	U	E	N	U	C
F	M	Z	V	W	R	P	F	G	K	D	C	M	N	D	F
F	R	L	E	R	A	I	I	V	X	N	Z	O	F	B	C
I	E	W	X	L	Y	D	L	T	E	J	I	J	B	D	N
C	L	G	U	O	A	G	Q	R	U	T	G	R	U	T	M
I	A	K	S	R	N	C	E	F	A	R	E	B	K	Z	Y
E	T	B	A	D	F	F	C	T	H	G	N	D	O	H	Q
N	I	P	P	B	N	A	N	O	A	Q	X	O	A	W	L
C	O	I	Z	O	N	E	S	N	U	X	H	W	V	C	L
Y	N	S	C	V	I	D	A	R	X	N	F	P	I	E	R
Y	S	Z	H	R	O	M	N	G	D	W	T	R	J	A	R
Z	H	X	O	H	T	L	Y	N	Z	T	J	A	W	B	P
Q	I	N	S	T	R	U	M	E	N	T	P	R	B	E	J
Z	P	M	E	A	S	U	R	E	W	E	Z	S	W	L	Z
V	J	O	P	E	R	A	T	I	O	N	S	H	D	M	E

PARADIGM
OPERATIONS
TRANSPARENCY
MANAGER
ORIENTATION
CONFERENCE
EFFICIENCY
TRAY
INSTRUMENT
MEASURE
ACCOUNTABLE
RELATIONSHIP
TURNOVER

OR/SPD Collaboration

The OR Today Live Conference

CALROAOTIBOLN
6 8 10 11 18

PGAHARICNMAGDE

CRNENECOFE
7 2

MRSUEAE
4

OIOAPRENTS
17 16

EFCIINCEFY

ACNBOAUTLCE
14 12

TRSNNCAAPERY
3

ATYR
1 13

RHOLINSEITAP
9

MAEGNAR

IETRNSNUMT

TEUOVRNR

ONOITARETIN
15

1 2 3 4 6 7 8 9 10 11 12 13 14 15 16 17 18

Discovering Your Why, Finding Your Voice, and Public Speaking

https://directory.libsyn.com/episode/index/id/6271852

Discovering Your Why

Finding Your Voice and Public Speaking

P	P	E	G	N	A	E	H	B	Z	I	U	F	D	V	P
S	H	X	P	Q	E	S	M	R	B	T	P	E	T	V	P
P	W	J	Y	R	D	D	E	P	V	Y	I	B	R	T	R
E	F	S	A	U	B	V	A	I	O	F	L	C	J	X	E
A	S	H	U	V	O	E	Z	D	I	W	H	H	L	H	S
K	S	Y	D	C	P	M	L	T	C	M	E	E	N	Y	E
I	U	A	S	G	C	U	R	I	E	H	T	R	R	Z	N
N	A	I	I	Z	O	E	R	K	E	K	P	T	W	A	T
G	D	T	I	M	C	Q	S	P	Q	V	S	C	P	U	A
F	K	U	N	U	P	P	N	S	O	U	E	P	O	D	T
Z	J	W	L	G	Q	O	K	H	D	S	P	J	Z	I	I
I	X	I	R	N	I	O	R	N	I	C	E	J	Q	E	O
V	U	P	K	S	W	Q	I	T	U	Y	D	O	S	N	N
Z	G	B	S	H	N	H	U	S	A	Y	M	C	W	C	S
U	D	A	Q	A	I	B	Y	G	F	N	A	E	R	E	I
P	P	B	X	P	Z	I	F	F	W	C	T	A	F	T	W

CERTIFIED
SPEAKING
VOICE
AUDIENCE
IMPORTANT
WHY
PRESENTATION
PURPOSE
SHARE
EMPOWER
DISCOVER
PASSION
INDUSTRY
BELIEVE
SUCCESS

Discovering Your Why

Finding Your Voice and Public Speaking

CETIRIEFD	☐☐☐☐☐☐☐☐☐	19
HYW	☐☐☐	12
DOIVESCR	☐☐☐☐☐☐☐☐	15
SIPKENAG	☐☐☐☐☐☐☐☐	
PTNOIAERTSEN	☐☐☐☐☐☐☐☐☐☐☐☐	2 16 10
POIASSN	☐☐☐☐☐☐☐	9
ICOEV	☐☐☐☐☐	6 13
POPUSRE	☐☐☐☐☐☐☐	
IUTRNSDY	☐☐☐☐☐☐☐☐	
ADICUENE	☐☐☐☐☐☐☐☐	14 4 7
HERSA	☐☐☐☐☐	17
BVIEELE	☐☐☐☐☐☐☐	1 3
ITARPNMOT	☐☐☐☐☐☐☐☐☐	
EOEPMWR	☐☐☐☐☐☐☐	
SCESUCS	☐☐☐☐☐☐☐	5

1	2	3	4	5	6	7		9	10		12	13	14	15	16	17	18	19
																	L	

An Industry in Transition: Stories from the Trenches

https://directory.libsyn.com/episode/index/id/9752219

An Industry in Transition

Stories from the Trenches

X	U	R	W	U	T	N	E	F	V	P	K	E	W	C	J
H	M	A	N	A	G	E	M	E	N	T	L	D	Y	K	Y
A	S	T	A	N	D	A	R	D	S	B	M	C	T	V	T
S	Y	X	I	W	E	S	L	F	I	S	A	A	I	N	N
E	T	H	N	B	D	P	E	S	I	R	W	A	X	C	E
G	V	N	M	F	R	R	I	J	E	T	G	R	E	O	M
N	S	Q	E	H	Y	V	F	L	Q	N	I	E	L	L	E
E	P	C	X	M	R	R	E	U	I	W	R	S	P	L	V
L	E	O	G	M	E	T	A	H	X	X	G	O	M	A	L
L	N	K	U	N	A	R	C	L	H	A	N	U	O	B	O
A	M	F	J	V	I	A	I	H	A	X	U	R	C	O	V
H	Z	J	I	K	E	K	A	U	O	S	G	C	A	R	N
C	P	T	K	T	O	W	L	Z	Q	V	T	E	W	A	I
U	O	W	B	F	U	K	T	A	N	E	T	S	Q	T	H
M	D	I	W	L	L	N	K	E	W	H	R	O	D	E	D
L	I	Q	N	O	I	T	A	M	R	O	F	N	I	I	Y

COMPLEXITY
RESOURCES
CARE
COLLABORATE
INVOLVEMENT

REQUIREMENTS
WALKING
MOTIVATE
CHALLENGES
MANAGEMENT

INFORMATION
TEACHING
VISIBLE
SALARY
STANDARDS

An Industry in Transition

Stories from the Trenches

CLIEPMOTXY ☐☐☐☐☐☐☐☐☐☐ (7)

RNTQEEEIMURS ☐☐☐☐☐☐☐☐☐☐☐☐ (20, 18)

IMNFOARIOTN ☐☐☐☐☐☐☐☐☐☐☐

RCUREESOS ☐☐☐☐☐☐☐☐☐ (19)

WINALKG ☐☐☐☐☐☐☐ (9, 10, 12)

TINECAHG ☐☐☐☐☐☐☐☐ (3)

ECAR ☐☐☐☐

MAOTTIVE ☐☐☐☐☐☐☐☐ (13)

VLIBISE ☐☐☐☐☐☐☐ (6, 2)

CLOORTABALE ☐☐☐☐☐☐☐☐☐☐☐ (1)

CANGHELELS ☐☐☐☐☐☐☐☐☐☐ (15)

SRAALY ☐☐☐☐☐☐

IVLMNOVENET ☐☐☐☐☐☐☐☐☐☐☐ (14, 11)

MNEAMNEGAT ☐☐☐☐☐☐☐☐☐☐ (17, 21)

SDATARDNS ☐☐☐☐☐☐☐☐☐ (4, 22)

1	2	3	4		6	7		9	10	11	12	13	14	15		17	18	19	20	21	22

Go Out Among the Hedges

The Place for Sterile Processing Leadership in Recruiting All-Stars

There is a story in the Bible about a man who was throwing a great feast (Luke 14). But when it came time for the festivities to begin, no one showed up. There were plenty of excuses to be heard, but the bottom line was this: after all the preparations had been made, the expected guests never came.

For many Sterile Processing leaders around the country, this is a familiar feeling. While we're not throwing great feasts, we are often busy making preparations -- requesting new positions, submitting staffing justifications, and finagling compensation to be just a little more competitive with our new hire wages. But when the time comes for our guests to arrive (hopefully stellar candidates looking for a career in Sterile Processing), the knock never comes on our door.

There are a number of persuasive reasons why this phenomenon is common in our field.

1. Pay grade is a problem.

For most facilities, entry-level Sterile Processing technicians come in around $12/hour. While this is not the $7+ minimum wage that comes with retail and food service positions, it is nowhere near the kind of compensation that will attract large numbers of bright, capable, career-oriented individuals -- on its own.

2. Clinical recruiting trumps support staff.

A reality in the hospital world is that the Recruiting department's time, money, and resources are focused in on finding and hiring high-quality clinical staff (RNs, Surgical Techs, etc.). Many recruiters have extensive experience hiring for nursing floors and the OR but are not in tune with the very different needs of Sterile Processing departments. By the time they finish with the clinical priorities, the candidate bucket for SPD is often dry.

3. We are out of sight and out of mind.

Not only is the physical location of the Sterile Processing department in the basement of the hospital, but it is often in the basement of a broader healthcare consciousness. Society knows about doctors and nurses, x-ray techs and anesthesiologists - but who ever heard of a sterilization tech? Is that, like, for people? Even with these excuses for why all-stars don't just show up at an SPD manager's door, there are a number of very practical things that department leaders can be doing to ensure their positions are filled with the best techs on the market.

- **Prepare more than just the seat cushions**.

Many leaders think the hard work is done once the final approval is received to hire an additional technician. They have an open chair, so why wouldn't someone amazing want to come sit in it? Often the answer has something to do with the aroma of the department as a whole. As corny as it sounds, does your department smell like excellence? Is it a place where employees not only feel challenged and fulfilled, but also where they feel like they have a critical role in pushing the department forward? No one wants to work at a place that feels more like a hamster wheel than a department that's actually going somewhere. It's up to Sterile Processing leaders to direct and cultivate this culture of growth and performance excellence in the department before the recruiting banquet ever starts.

- **Take the reins and go out among the hedges.**

If you realize that the traditional "approved & waiting" recruiting model isn't meeting your needs, take a proactive approach to finding high-quality candidates yourself. Find out when the local graduate schools have their job fairs and set up a booth. Reach out to nursing schools to post job openings on their employment boards. Partner with local refugee/immigrant placement agencies who often have candidates with extensive medical experience just looking for a way back into healthcare. What you can't do is continue to wait, and hope that your next high performer just wanders in off the street. Is it your job to do all this? Maybe not. Does it make your job a lot easier in the future? You bet it does.

- **Clean out the rusty pipes and enjoy the rain.**

Once your department culture is in place (one that rewards high performers and lays out opportunity for growth) and the proactive recruiting pipelines have been opened into your local community -- the initial trickle of hard-won candidates will eventually turn into a regular downpour. Birds of a professional feather like to flock together. High-performers want to work among other high-performers. If you can do the difficult work of breaking out of the rusty recruiting model of "sit & wait," the network of all-star Sterile Processing techs will eventually begin recruiting themselves. The pipeline will always require tending and you will often have more candidates than you have positions available to hire -- but what a terrific problem to have!
Plan the banquet, then go out among the hedges and bring 'em to the feast.

Sterile Processing Certification
The CBSPD Spotlight (Part 2)

https://directory.libsyn.com/episode/index/id/6826727

Sterile Processing Certification

The CBSPD Spotlight

N	J	R	J	H	I	K	Q	M	O	C	E	H	A	F	Y
O	F	N	L	A	I	T	N	E	D	E	R	C	B	T	Q
I	D	Z	E	N	D	O	S	C	O	P	E	M	W	F	N
T	R	U	T	N	E	T	E	P	M	O	C	L	C	O	W
A	J	E	P	A	V	M	D	T	T	R	G	T	I	E	A
I	T	H	N	X	P	A	R	E	A	V	Y	T	F	M	Y
C	D	E	Z	E	H	D	A	B	Y	T	A	C	P	D	S
O	X	N	S	Y	W	P	O	H	E	Z	S	S	N	A	P
S	K	K	Q	T	V	A	B	X	I	N	A	C	U	P	H
S	O	J	R	K	L	S	L	N	E	L	E	N	Y	P	Q
A	L	A	T	T	X	W	A	M	D	S	W	F	O	Q	O
O	L	M	Z	Q	N	G	G	A	P	X	N	I	I	N	E
V	T	K	M	T	R	D	K	X	H	C	N	E	B	T	K
R	Q	V	E	O	W	Q	Q	E	H	T	U	C	C	U	S
F	C	S	K	I	L	L	S	A	S	R	U	S	I	I	V
T	K	Q	X	L	N	O	I	T	A	C	U	D	E	K	L

EXAM	EDUCATION	STATE
BOARD	ORGANIZATION	LICENSE
ASSOCIATION	TEST	SKILLS
ENDOSCOPE	RENEWAL	POINTS
COMPETENT	CREDENTIAL	BENEFITS

Sterile Processing Certification

The CBSPD Spotlight

MEXA

EUADOICTN (13, 2, 18, 7)

ATTES

ADROB (19, 3)

OTIIROAGAZNN (12, 16)

LESNCIE (15)

ACTIOISAOSN (11)

ESTT

SILKLS (4, 20)

EOCDNPOSE (21, 9)

REANEWL

PNOTIS (17)

CENMTEPOT

CIETAERNDL (8, 5)

BNIEETFS (6)

Q																			
1	2	3	4	5	6	7	8	9	11	12	13	15	16	17	18	19	20	21	

Surveying the Surveyor, What You Need to Know (Part 1)

https://directory.libsyn.com/episode/index/id/6826734

Surveying the Surveyor

What You Need to Know

K	Z	I	X	E	Z	N	X	T	E	I	C	K	Y	T	P
X	S	Z	P	Z	Q	M	I	C	E	G	V	Q	C	W	U
R	Q	U	Y	G	U	P	N	P	E	A	N	X	N	A	C
O	E	J	O	V	D	E	F	C	A	X	M	W	E	I	O
D	C	W	K	V	I	A	N	M	M	F	W	J	I	P	N
X	F	L	S	R	R	A	E	T	E	Q	Q	S	C	R	V
A	K	D	E	N	I	E	G	L	L	Q	T	X	I	Y	E
X	A	P	A	L	A	Q	N	T	O	G	E	P	F	E	R
X	X	B	P	E	W	B	P	M	K	K	Z	O	E	V	S
E	B	M	T	C	E	P	S	E	R	M	N	N	D	R	A
J	O	D	N	D	G	C	D	E	N	I	A	R	T	U	T
C	N	O	I	T	A	T	I	D	E	R	C	C	A	S	I
R	B	A	C	K	G	R	O	U	N	D	F	J	Q	M	O
V	Y	E	G	N	E	L	L	A	H	C	W	M	K	P	N
L	L	O	F	W	W	N	O	I	T	S	E	U	Q	M	K
A	H	R	W	E	X	Q	O	P	X	R	C	N	T	J	B

SURVEY
ANSWER
ACCREDITATION
COMPLIANCE
CONVERSATION
BACKGROUND
EXPERIENCE
TRAINED
NERVOUS
CHALLENGE
QUESTION
DEFICIENCY
TEAM
LEAD
RESPECT

Surveying the Surveyor

What You Need to Know

SEVURY ☐☐☐☐☐☐ (3)

BOGUKCRNAD ☐☐☐☐☐☐☐☐☐☐

QOUISETN ☐☐☐☐☐☐☐☐ (12 13 17 18)

AWESNR ☐☐☐☐☐☐ (2 4 14)

ENIPEXRCEE ☐☐☐☐☐☐☐☐☐☐

DCEEFCIINY ☐☐☐☐☐☐☐☐☐☐

AOIAIRECCTDTN ☐☐☐☐☐☐☐☐☐☐☐☐☐ (16)

TNEAIRD ☐☐☐☐☐☐☐ (6 1)

MTEA ☐☐☐☐ (5)

CAPONCIMLE ☐☐☐☐☐☐☐☐☐☐ (19)

NUOEVRS ☐☐☐☐☐☐☐

ADEL ☐☐☐☐

CSORNOAVIETN ☐☐☐☐☐☐☐☐☐☐☐☐ (8)

CLNELAGHE ☐☐☐☐☐☐☐☐☐ (9)

RCEESPT ☐☐☐☐☐☐☐ (15 10)

1 2 3 4 5 6   8 9 10   12 13 14 15 16 17 18 19

Expertise vs Accreditation – Challenges to the Surveying Process

https://directory.libsyn.com/episode/index/id/6916757

Expertise vs Accreditation

Challenges to the Surveying Process

F	D	G	U	I	D	E	L	I	N	E	S	M	S	I	K
T	C	A	W	E	A	K	N	E	S	S	E	T	G	G	R
L	O	L	J	S	M	J	J	B	H	W	C	D	O	O	E
F	R	V	T	B	U	A	Q	T	J	U	S	Z	T	R	F
J	R	S	O	Z	E	F	G	S	D	T	Z	A	V	I	E
K	E	R	U	B	D	N	V	O	C	R	R	A	Y	N	R
X	C	I	P	N	E	W	R	A	E	T	T	Y	O	S	E
S	T	W	B	R	P	P	F	I	S	Q	K	I	P	P	N
U	I	X	T	N	A	P	G	I	F	K	T	N	E	E	C
R	O	S	I	T	R	T	N	H	Z	S	O	R	H	C	E
V	N	W	R	I	T	I	N	G	E	N	A	P	I	T	F
E	K	B	V	N	M	R	M	U	Z	H	Z	O	J	I	M
Y	G	C	W	D	E	T	Q	H	S	I	X	V	K	O	L
O	J	N	A	I	N	O	Q	P	D	J	J	H	O	N	R
R	H	C	F	I	T	N	R	L	S	R	F	O	Q	C	M
E	I	X	C	B	K	E	J	P	K	K	D	Q	U	N	V

STRENGTH
GUIDELINES
QUESTION
INSPECTION
SURVEYOR
WEAKNESS
CORRECTION
REFERENCE
PRODUCTS
SHARE
FACTS
WRITING
ADMINISTRATOR
DEPARTMENT
TONE

Expertise vs Accreditation

Challenges to the Surveying Process

STTGRNEH

1 12 11

WASEEKNS

5 18

TCFSA

14 4

GDNEEIIULS

CRITOOCREN

16 2

WITNRIG

QEOIUTSN

17

REECNREFE

AOTAMDNISIRTR

7

IICONPESTN

3 8

PUTODRCS

DNRMTEPAET

15

SVORUEYR

ESHAR

ENTO

10

1 2 3 4 5 7 8 10 11 12 14 15 16 17 18

The $50 Billion Dollar Opportunity Re-Thinking the Economics of Sterile Processing

https://directory.libsyn.com/episode/index/id/9303893

The $50 Billion Dollar Opportunity

Re-Thinking the Economics of Sterile Processing

L	C	M	W	Q	E	C	O	N	O	M	I	C	S	Q	M
T	U	Q	J	A	U	N	W	S	Y	C	F	U	R	L	B
E	T	O	Y	V	S	U	D	T	U	N	U	S	E	D	Z
W	F	Q	X	E	H	T	I	Y	E	Q	D	J	P	B	C
D	B	W	T	T	C	X	E	L	X	G	E	G	R	A	O
Z	C	Y	W	E	E	A	I	P	N	G	L	N	O	K	M
V	Y	O	A	L	C	K	R	I	Q	T	A	B	F	Y	P
I	R	O	P	P	A	H	S	E	T	Y	Y	E	E	E	E
G	Y	M	A	S	T	S	N	I	E	M	S	N	S	L	N
V	O	Y	U	N	E	U	O	I	B	R	O	U	S	G	S
C	O	R	U	C	S	P	R	D	C	M	K	W	I	F	A
X	K	X	O	Y	U	H	K	N	Z	I	I	C	O	S	T
K	F	R	A	E	W	N	J	O	O	A	A	G	N	W	I
L	P	C	G	Z	V	H	B	C	S	V	X	N	A	O	O
M	I	S	S	I	N	G	O	A	H	N	E	M	L	W	N
O	J	N	C	N	S	Z	U	U	M	Y	C	R	G	B	W

WASTE
UNUSED
COMPLEXITY
CAREER
MONEY
TURNOVER
COST
DELAYS
GROWTH
TECHNICIAN
PROCESSING
COMPENSATION
MISSING
ECONOMICS
PROFESSIONAL

The $50 Billion Dollar Opportunity

Re-Thinking the Economics of Sterile Processing

Scrambled word	Boxes	Numbered boxes
TWESA	5	10
TRVOENUR	8	4, 16, 18, 19, 21
PERNSCSOIG	10	8
USNEUD	6	15, 3
OTCS	4	14
CPNMTOEOASIN	12	
CLXOEMITPY	10	9
DLAYES	6	
MNISSIG	7	
CEEARR	6	1, 20
GTROWH	6	
ENMOICCOS	9	2, 17
NMYOE	5	
THIICNACEN	10	5
PAINSOERSOFL	12	11, 6

1	2	3	4	5	6

8	9	10	11	12
				F

14	15	16	17	18	19	20	21

High Marks & High Standards
Compliant Reprocessing of
Reusable Medical Devices

https://directory.libsyn.com/episode/index/id/9752219

High Marks & High Standards

Compliant Reprocessing of Reusable Medical Devices

S	J	R	J	Z	H	B	H	P	B	X	I	N	J	T	N
X	C	L	O	G	R	U	F	F	R	R	Z	O	X	B	Q
F	L	O	C	V	O	L	U	N	T	A	R	Y	N	J	L
O	N	F	M	Q	I	H	L	R	H	V	C	T	V	N	E
S	N	R	M	P	U	N	O	Z	Y	C	N	T	B	K	M
T	Z	Z	E	A	L	Y	C	B	M	O	T	D	I	E	P
A	W	F	U	G	E	E	O	E	I	C	R	A	S	C	R
N	C	G	Y	V	U	B	T	T	N	A	V	E	T	W	E
D	K	C	R	H	K	L	A	E	Z	T	N	M	P	W	S
A	F	U	U	C	A	M	A	A	J	I	I	Z	D	F	E
R	S	B	E	R	R	O	H	T	L	V	H	V	I	Q	N
D	E	X	M	O	A	O	P	E	O	H	A	Y	E	R	T
Y	A	N	F	O	I	T	D	T	V	R	X	K	J	A	A
W	R	N	F	B	O	I	E	S	S	M	Y	H	W	L	B
K	I	E	N	S	U	Z	S	R	V	F	Y	T	K	B	L
I	O	C	Q	G	J	C	K	Y	L	J	D	C	E	X	E

STANDARD
PRACTICE
VOLUNTARY
PRESENTABLE
GUIDELINES
INFORMATION
COMPLETE
REGULATORY
INCENTIVE
SURVEYOR
ACCURATE
BIOHAZARD

High Marks & High Standards

Compliant Reprocessing of Reusable Medical Devices

SANRTDAD

GEDLUNIEIS
6 7

RIEDOCAMNTOEMN
3

IVINCETNE

PCIARCTE
10 8 15

IRMAFOINTON

SVORUEYR
1 17

VROAUNLTY

CPOEMTLE
2

AUATCRCE
13

PSANBELETRE
14 5

ADAIIOTCRETCN
12 16

RTOGARULEY
11

BRAAIHOZD

DONIEIANMATTCON

1 2 3 5 6 7 8 10 11 12 13 14 15 16 17

Sterile Processing Service Excellence

5 Tips to Become the Chick-fil-A of Your Surgical Team

Although a large number of Sterile Processing departments across the country still bear the name Central "Service", many still deal with the daily challenges of excelling in the area of customer service. Sterile Processing is a high stress job, with quality expectations of zero errors, coupled with grueling time constraints and a customer pool that is often not the gentlest communicators of their needs. And believe it or not, your local Chick-fil-A has the exact same challenges -- but they have found a way to both dominate the competition and please their customers. Here are five tips for your Sterile Processing team that could help your department mirror the Chick-fil-A customer service flare:

1. Hire with your customer in mind

You know your customers better than anyone else, so be intentional about hiring SPD techs according to your overarching department emphasis on customer service. Include questions in your interview process about how the candidate has handled an irate customer in the past or ask them to describe a time when they had to communicate complex information to someone outside their department. This goes beyond the typical focus on brains (technical knowledge) and brawn (physical ability to do the job), and instead, gets to the heart of their ability to be a service-oriented technician. Chick-fil-a hires like this, and so should we.

2. Set the standards and train accordingly

If you walk into any Chick-fil-a in the country and tell one of their employees "Thank you" their response will be the same in Ft. Lauderdale, Florida as it is in Austin, Texas, ...a simple, "My pleasure." As quaint is it may sound, this kind of standardized language of customer service is critical for cultivating the larger cultural service-standards of your department. Whatever areas you want to focus on -- be it how you answer the phone, "Thank for calling Sterile Processing, my name is John. How may I assist you today?" or a generalized script for dealing with angry physicians -- you must utilize your training period to inculcate these behaviors into your team. No one comes out of the womb saying "My pleasure" in response to everything, but no one at Chick-fil-a works the front register without it. Our expectations in Sterile Processing should be just as high.

3. Integrate "Second-Mile Service" into Daily Expectations

It's one thing to have a quiet OR for the day, which often means that at least nothing huge is going wrong. But even if every case today has all the instruments it needs to go smoothly, that doesn't necessarily mean your customer base is being wowed. What can move someone from being a satisfied customer to a raving fan is what Chick-fil-A calls "Second-Mile Service." It's not an earth-shattering concept, but it's often overlooked in the busy hustle and bustle of hospital life.

You must integrate a daily expectation of going beyond what your customer is asking for and key in on the secondary service opportunities that will communicate to them your genuine care for their quality experience. Nothing resonates more with an OR manager than the words, "Let me take care of that for you." And then do it excellently.

4. Grow your Own Leaders

I'm not sure how well-documented or structured this practice is from the corporate level of Chick-fil-A, but it is commonplace for their stores to promote from within. That concept is not unique to their organization, but they do it very often and very well. The reason this impacts growth in service excellence is that every leader who is promoted in that organization has demonstrated the ability to serve customers well and a commitment to keeping that value central to their broader philosophy of work. If you want a department that will continue to improve in the area of customer service, promote those high-performing, service-oriented techs right in your midst.

5. Share the excitement and believe in your mission

No one dresses up like giant tacos or quarter-pounders every year to get free food from the Taco Bells and McDonalds of the world. But how many pictures of little babies and grown men dressed up like cows have you seen splashed across social media during one of Chick-fil-A's "Cow Appreciation Days"...?

Or did you know that hundreds of people campout at every grand-opening of a Chick-fil-a store across the country? The company creates this kind of excitement among its customers because their team believes in their mission. A quote that you'll see posted in most of their restaurant lobbies reads, "Food is essential to life. Therefore, make it good." As a Sterile Processing department, you can be just as excited about your mission -- and that excitement cannot help but be spread to your customers. Someone once said, "If you set yourself on fire with passion, folks will come for miles to watch you burn." When your passion for service excellence is what you become known for around the hospital, all that's left is to continue to fan the flame.

So, here's to having your beverage "refreshed", your order delivered to your table, and your every concerned greeted by a smiling face and a coupon for a free chicken sandwich. Take that model and serve your surgical team with the same level of excellence.

W. Hank Balch ©

Policies & Patients
Insights on Explant Reprocessing

https://directory.libsyn.com/episode/index/id/9832229

Policies & Patients

Insights on Explant Reprocessing

Z	L	Z	S	I	B	E	A	K	E	D	X	W	K	S	R
J	O	C	U	P	F	Y	I	C	E	L	B	P	G	L	J
S	R	G	L	S	P	B	N	U	X	N	E	L	C	A	E
T	P	V	T	T	R	A	N	S	P	O	R	T	O	A	N
M	G	A	T	H	R	X	M	X	L	H	I	N	N	O	F
A	P	X	T	U	B	F	L	H	A	I	M	B	T	R	D
N	U	C	S	I	A	I	W	A	N	R	P	L	A	E	H
U	T	N	L	I	E	L	O	U	T	G	L	Y	M	K	W
F	I	U	Y	E	F	N	X	H	O	U	A	W	I	P	E
A	W	O	E	W	A	I	T	C	A	R	N	V	N	T	I
C	C	C	H	L	J	N	Y	X	K	Z	T	H	A	B	H
T	A	Y	R	S	Y	C	I	S	L	C	A	C	T	T	T
U	T	L	X	V	I	Y	I	N	C	P	U	R	E	S	F
R	I	T	U	L	M	R	E	W	G	D	K	F	D	L	X
E	X	N	O	K	L	I	G	L	E	P	L	N	C	Y	W
R	T	P	U	Q	B	I	O	B	U	R	D	E	N	A	X

- IMPLANT
- MANUFACTURER
- INSURANCE
- EDUCATE
- BIOBURDEN
- EXPLANT
- CONTAMINATED
- CLEANING
- TRANSPORT
- RISK
- PATIENT
- BIOHAZARD
- POLICY
- BLOOD

Policies & Patients

Insights on Explant Reprocessing

ILANMPT _ _ _ _ _ _ _

EAXPNLT _ 15 16 _ _ _ _

PNIATET _ _ _ _ _ _ _

MEUCTFAUANRR _ _ _ _ _ _ _ _ _ _ 2 _

CAAONNMTTEID _ 5 _ _ _ _ _ _ _ 20 _ _

BAZRHIAOD _ _ _ _ _ _ 18 _ _

IRACUNSNE _ 19 9 _ 1 _ 11 _ _

CNLNIEAG _ 17 7 _ _ _ _ 12

PLICOY 3 _ _ _ 6 _

ECDATUE _ _ _ _ _ _ 14

TONPARSRT _ _ _ _ 21 _ _ 4 _

ITNISTNUORCS _ _ 8 _ _ _ _ _ _ _ _ _

DOOBL _ _ _ _ _

BUIEDOBRN _ 10 _ _ _ _ _ _ _

KRIS _ _ _ _

1	2	3	4	5	6	7	8	9	10	11	12	14	15	16	17	18	19	20	21

Higher Education
Collaborating With Technical Colleges to Improve Sterile Processing

https://directory.libsyn.com/episode/index/id/10419818

Higher Education

Collaborating With Technical Colleges to Improve Sterile Processing

E	X	P	E	R	I	E	N	C	E	Y	N	P	L	I	N
R	Y	P	V	S	N	O	R	U	N	H	F	Y	I	D	K
F	K	R	L	K	C	E	R	O	B	D	X	T	H	I	V
W	G	Q	T	F	G	H	I	V	P	E	E	J	O	O	M
Q	I	T	Z	E	R	T	O	I	P	G	C	C	D	L	T
J	U	N	L	V	A	E	H	O	Q	R	Q	F	A	R	T
F	R	L	S	C	H	S	C	S	L	E	V	C	M	N	Y
O	O	V	U	T	R	O	L	R	S	E	I	F	E	Q	B
C	P	D	Q	E	R	X	S	R	U	N	J	D	L	M	U
T	E	D	D	M	Z	U	U	P	H	I	U	O	A	L	M
O	A	A	K	U	D	O	C	C	I	T	T	M	X	L	V
N	E	D	B	I	C	K	E	T	S	T	P	I	Q	Q	K
L	P	U	D	W	P	T	V	A	O	O	A	Z	N	I	K
O	T	Y	Y	G	K	U	Y	Z	T	R	U	L	T	G	I
T	V	K	P	B	P	R	O	G	R	A	M	J	F	C	T
G	Y	Q	L	A	Z	G	R	A	D	U	A	T	E	S	P

PROGRAM
TECHNICAL
LEADERSHIP
INSTRUCTOR
COLLEGE
EDUCATION
RECRUITING
GRADUATES
EXPERIENCE
COURSE
SCHOOL
HOSPITAL
DEGREE
STUDENT

Higher Education

Collaborating With Technical Colleges

EAIDTOCUN
12 20

SOCOHL
4

TCHACEINL
3 23

RIINRECUTG
21

HTOISAPL
14 6 8 9

LERADIESHP
2 13

GUREADATS
1

DGREEE
22

ITUCTNROSR
19 7 15

EEXPICRENE
18

SDNUTET
11 5

IPRMEOMENVT
24

CLEOGLE
16

CRSUOE

1 2 3 4 5 6 7 8 9 | 11 12 13 14 15 16 | 18 19 20 21 22 23 24

Certified Quality
Taking Sterile Processing Surveys to the Next Level

https://directory.libsyn.com/episode/index/id/10681487

Certified Quality

Taking Sterile Processing Surveys to the Next Level

O	R	G	A	N	I	Z	A	T	I	O	N	H	G	U	C
S	S	X	D	H	O	S	P	I	T	A	L	W	G	W	A
N	A	G	G	F	W	U	E	T	P	P	V	W	Z	S	Z
S	P	E	D	L	E	A	D	E	R	S	H	I	P	C	Q
H	T	R	M	F	K	X	M	G	O	M	O	W	P	I	J
D	C	A	A	K	A	Q	O	G	G	H	K	K	F	B	B
E	W	O	N	C	Z	N	O	L	R	P	T	Z	W	C	Y
P	Y	O	M	D	T	B	A	S	A	W	A	I	W	T	L
A	I	A	K	P	A	I	S	L	M	K	A	K	I	I	I
R	L	Y	O	A	L	R	C	D	Y	V	C	L	X	J	N
T	I	R	K	J	Y	I	D	E	W	S	A	O	A	Y	I
M	I	J	P	U	T	N	A	I	A	U	I	Q	O	D	H
E	U	E	G	L	M	X	C	N	Q	K	M	S	C	B	O
N	B	N	S	R	E	P	R	O	C	E	S	S	I	N	G
T	E	P	I	K	M	A	N	A	G	E	M	E	N	T	H
P	H	Q	C	O	N	S	I	S	T	E	N	C	Y	Y	Z

QUALITY
CONSISTENCY
REPROCESSING
DEPARTMENT
PRACTICE
MANAGEMENT
HOSPITAL
LEADERSHIP
PROGRAM
STANDARD
ANALYSIS
COMPLIANCE
ORGANIZATION

Certified Quality

Taking Sterile Processing Surveys to the Next Level

Word	Numbered boxes
QLIATUY	4, 21
MNAENEGMAT	9, 13
SAARTNDD	
CCSONINTSEY	19, 10
CIECFATOIITRN	17, 18, 6
HIOSTAPL	23, 3
AYIALNSS	24
ARODCACIIETTN	5, 8, 1, 22
RESNEPCRISOG	12, 2
LAEISEHDRP	14
CALICMNPOE	7
DNATEMEPRT	15
PAGRORM	
OGTAIRAOZINN	16
PCITACRE	20

1 2 3 4 5 6 7 8 9 10   12 13 14 15 16 17 18 19 20 21 22 23 24

Insights from South Africa Sterile Processing Perspectives and Regional Challenges

https://directory.libsyn.com/episode/index/id/10830890

Insights from South Africa

Sterile Processing Perspectives and Regional Challenges

W	M	J	S	F	U	R	V	F	T	S	L	D	D	B	J
X	C	R	J	S	W	H	Y	T	Q	T	E	B	N	E	X
X	N	E	D	A	R	B	R	C	Y	B	M	U	Q	L	W
G	Y	P	Q	P	F	O	T	K	J	R	S	S	S	H	N
V	L	R	A	P	A	F	N	U	T	D	D	S	B	S	T
E	A	O	Z	T	Q	Y	U	D	B	A	R	A	L	S	I
D	N	C	B	R	B	Q	O	L	S	E	W	R	E	X	V
E	I	E	S	A	I	O	C	N	D	A	E	G	P	K	T
I	P	S	C	F	L	Y	O	A	S	G	N	C	A	Y	Q
F	O	S	P	N	Y	I	E	H	I	E	D	T	T	M	V
I	Z	I	L	B	T	L	E	O	L	J	H	I	L	I	A
L	Q	N	G	U	P	R	N	L	K	H	L	U	L	C	M
A	F	G	L	Y	S	A	A	M	J	A	S	L	I	T	I
U	O	O	A	S	L	H	Y	I	U	H	U	R	J	C	Y
Q	S	U	E	W	C	G	R	Q	W	S	F	E	M	T	W
Y	Y	T	E	C	H	N	I	C	I	A	N	S	D	Q	N

AFRICA
QUALIFIED
SOLUTIONS
LEADERS
WASHERS
REGIONAL
QUALITY
ISSUES
GLOBAL
CHALLENGES
COUNTRY
TECHNICIANS
REPROCESSING

Insights from South Africa

Sterile Processing Perspectives and Regional Challenges

Scrambled word	Boxes	Numbered boxes
ARCFIA	6	4th: 9; 6th: 7
PVEICSRETEPS	12	
RNEGIAOL	8	3rd: 19; 4th: 18; 6th: 2
CEEGNLHALS	10	2nd: 20; 7th: 16; 10th: 22
QAIIELFUD	9	
CNSOAIOMEPTN	12	6th: 6; 8th: 12; 9th: 3; 12th: 11
QAIUTLY	7	6th: 21
CUTORNY	7	5th: 8
SNTOUOILS	9	2nd: 10
ISUESS	6	
TCCNIENHIAS	11	6th: 1; 8th: 15
LAREEDS	7	1st: 13; 2nd: 4
GBAOLL	6	
RPRSESNECOIG	12	4th: 5
WHERASS	7	3rd: 17

1	2	3	4	5	6	7	8	9	10	11	12	13		15	16	17	18	19	20	21	22

The Good, the Bad, and the Ugly
What to Look For In a Medical Device Sales Representative

https://directory.libsyn.com/episode/index/id/10887881

The Good, the Bad, and the Ugly

What to Look For In a Medical Device Sales Representative

P	N	O	I	T	A	C	I	N	U	M	M	O	C	X	M
T	E	H	D	H	V	X	X	C	S	G	S	G	P	P	N
S	C	K	L	X	R	R	A	T	I	T	M	K	I	H	O
N	I	Y	I	P	W	S	R	I	C	R	C	Q	H	Y	I
O	V	Z	R	K	I	E	L	U	B	U	W	Q	S	S	T
I	R	K	I	O	P	M	D	L	S	Y	J	F	N	I	A
T	E	V	U	X	T	O	K	T	I	Y	K	Z	O	C	C
A	S	C	E	A	R	I	O	G	T	K	X	P	I	I	U
T	E	G	A	P	N	M	R	I	B	K	S	Y	T	A	D
C	V	X	L	Q	E	P	X	R	R	L	B	P	A	N	E
E	I	F	H	R	X	E	G	A	E	Y	L	T	L	S	S
P	R	Y	S	G	L	H	J	A	X	T	C	S	E	M	K
X	D	I	J	P	L	P	N	L	W	U	A	C	R	M	L
E	O	X	M	U	A	G	J	S	C	L	R	M	V	P	F
G	Y	O	E	L	J	S	E	L	E	C	D	T	Q	K	G
T	C	M	L	X	M	Z	D	S	A	J	P	Y	F	N	I

SERVICE
TERRITORY
SKILLS
CUSTOMER
DRIVE
PRODUCTS
EXPERTS
COMMUNICATION
RELATIONSHIP
COMPLEXITY
SALES
EDUCATION
PHYSICIAN
EXPECTATIONS

The Good, the Bad, and the Ugly

What to Look For In a Medical Device Sales Representative

Scrambled word	Boxes	Numbers under boxes
REATETNRPSVEIE	14	box 2: 13; box 6: 14; box 11: 20
SCEIRVE	7	box 1: 19; box 2: 7
PUROCTDS	8	box 5: 2
LEASS	5	
TTRREORIY	9	box 7: 5; box 8: 18
EREXTPS	7	
EODATUCIN	9	box 8: 11
SLKILS	6	
CUICTOAIOMNMN	13	box 1: 1; box 4: 12; box 8: 10
COMSTEUR	8	box 3: 3; box 6: 6; box 8: 8
RTAISNELIOHP	12	box 5: 4
PICAYISHN	9	box 5: 17
EIVDR	5	
CTPIMXLOEY	10	
EETPINXAOTCS	12	

													F				
1	2	3	4	5	6	7	8	10	11	12	13	14	16	17	18	19	20

Cultivating your Team: How to "Grow Your Own" Sterile Processing Leaders

Where do future sterile processing leaders hang out? Is there some local hole-in-the-wall where they congregate after a long day's work? Are they currently walking around town with shirts that proclaim, "I Want to Supervise -- Please Hire Me"?

If you've been in the Sterile Processing world long enough, you know that finding stellar leaders, when you need them, is one of the hardest parts of leading a department forward. It's not uncommon for CS departments to go through multiple managers and supervisors over a 5-year period, with no consistent theme for the kinds of leaders they are looking for.

In this post, I'd like to argue that some of your best candidates for future SPD leadership can (and should) come from inside your own department. Here are some reasons why this is the case, and how to make it happen in your own backyard...

1. Hire frontline techs with the leadership in mind

Michael Dell once said, "If you're the smartest person in the room, you're in the wrong room." As you interview for entry level SPD tech positions, always be thinking about what inherent qualities this person has for future leadership opportunities -- and, if you can, try to hire folks who are smarter than you. This will mean that you look for more qualities in a potential candidate than just the ones that will make them a high performing tech. Just because someone is a great tech, does not mean they would make a great SPD leader. Hire those candidates who demonstrate personal accountability, ability to collaborate with diverse teams, willingness to accept additional responsibilities as they Learn the job, and other big-picture skills that make them stand out from the average worker-bee. They are harder to find, but worth their weight in leadership gold.

2. Shake up the traditional expectations for department responsibilities

So, you've got some staff who are standing out as potential future leaders (either because you hired or inherited them). What's next? This is where leadership growth becomes really fun. The traditional model of promote and pray, leaves departments open to the dangers of wanting to give opportunities to hard-working techs -- but not having given them the prior experiences necessary for them to excel in their new leadership role. One way to prep these potential leaders is to intentionally flatten out the day-to-day responsibilities of department coordinators, supervisors, and managers in order to give frontline technicians exposure to leadership right where they're at. This could mean doing simple things like giving workshops on how to create staffing schedules and allowing various techs to work with current supervisors in creating next week's schedule. Or, it could mean alternating responsibility for attending daily safety meetings with hospital leadership. Any responsibility than can be shared, should be shared -- with a long-term vision for equipping your team to take future leadership opportunities.

3. Apply the "miracle-grow" of abundant involvement in leadership life

If you want your team to be ready to step into a promotion without encountering a crippling learning curve, do your best to involve them in as much of the big-picture planning as you can. If you're having an important meeting with instrument repair vendors, ask one of your techs to come along and listen to the dialog. Not only will they gain a broader perspective on the overall department, but you can then follow-up with them after the meeting on how/why you interacted with the vendors the way you did. If you're reporting to the infection control or quality steering committee, bring along a tech to give them a picture of the higher-level of accountability that SPD leaders experience. The more opportunity they have to learn the language of leadership and come to understand the department culture you are operating out of, the more likely they will be ready when the time comes for promotions.

4. Go out of your way to plant your people

Although this is a cursory point, it's still key to creating this kind of synergy of people and potential: as a Sterile Processing leader, you must go out of your way to find opportunities for your team to grow. This means soliciting genuine answers to the question of "This time next year, where do you want to be?" And be prepared when the answers are not Sterile Processing related. I have folks who work for me who want to do everything from enroll in nursing school to start their own business. If you will demonstrate your commitment to their future plans through concrete, proactive mentorship, you will get employees who trust you to be looking out for their best interests when you approach them with leadership opportunities within your department. If your team knows that you're not just trying to 'plug a hole', but are instead developing them as individuals, you will see many of them jump at the opportunity on the table.

5. Impacting growth by cultivating it

Finally, while promoting from within is not always the best-case scenario for Sterile Processing teams (for instance, if the department is in need of a complete culture shift), doing so can have all kinds of benefits for your department

First and foremost, if you are able to grow your own leaders, this implies that the new leader will be stepping in with the same overall culture and goals as the previous leader. This level of stability is critical for many departments to overcome the natural anxieties of a changing of the guard. Secondly, hiring from within gives confirmation and credence to the leadership growth initiatives that you have already put in place and encourages other potential leaders to continue their pursuit of career growth. Once you build this "grow your own" track record as a department, you will begin to see the impact in your recruiting pool -- high performers want to work at a place where growth potential is real, not just pie-in-the-sky. It's just like that little snowball at the top of a mountain, the longer it rolls, the larger it gets.

Simply put, if you can hire well, engage your technicians with various opportunities for responsibility, and do your job as their growth-advocate, you will wake up one day to a field of future leaders ripe for the harvest. You may have more leaders than you know what to do with, but that's a heck of a problem to have.

The Human Connection Networking and Success in Sterile Processing

https://directory.libsyn.com/episode/index/id/12023738

The Human Connection

Networking and Success in Sterile Processing

G	K	N	O	W	L	E	D	G	E	N	G	W	L	M	L
E	S	M	K	R	I	W	E	V	T	C	A	Q	O	B	S
T	W	R	H	P	Q	O	U	K	R	R	H	D	L	Z	W
P	E	E	T	Y	K	D	X	J	U	O	C	F	T	U	B
R	K	T	W	H	T	D	H	L	N	O	T	E	F	B	W
O	A	S	O	B	V	I	A	P	N	K	E	N	D	D	E
F	D	O	R	U	X	N	N	N	X	E	R	L	E	Y	D
E	E	P	G	B	O	E	E	U	Y	Y	T	P	D	M	U
S	X	M	N	S	T	C	V	B	T	P	S	W	E	T	C
S	S	I	R	W	T	R	D	C	O	R	F	V	N	K	A
I	Q	E	O	I	E	F	K	S	D	C	O	E	I	N	T
O	P	R	O	E	G	U	I	A	C	H	L	P	J	H	I
N	K	N	R	Q	V	T	R	Z	H	A	R	L	P	X	O
A	F	A	A	U	I	R	X	K	T	A	G	S	W	O	N
L	C	Q	L	O	G	Y	T	B	N	O	I	S	S	A	P
S	V	L	N	S	U	H	A	K	Q	X	O	X	N	D	Z

MENTOR
CAREER
PERSONAL
NETWORK
EDUCATION

CONNECTION
TALENT
GROWTH
STRETCH
KNOWLEDGE

OPPORTUNITY
PROFESSIONAL
IMPOSTER
POSITION
PASSION

The Human Connection

Networking and Success in Sterile Processing

MNTOER ☐☐☐☐☐☐ (2)

CTOCNNIOEN ☐☐☐☐☐☐☐☐☐☐

ONPPTIRUTOY ☐☐☐☐☐☐☐☐☐☐☐ (3, 1)

CEERAR ☐☐☐☐☐☐

TENLAT ☐☐☐☐☐☐

PAOSFSIONREL ☐☐☐☐☐☐☐☐☐☐☐☐ (6, 11, 15)

PSENAORL ☐☐☐☐☐☐☐☐ (16, 7)

GOWTRH ☐☐☐☐☐☐ (4, 8, 9)

ITSEMOPR ☐☐☐☐☐☐☐☐ (13)

NTREWOK ☐☐☐☐☐☐☐ (14)

SCTRTEH ☐☐☐☐☐☐☐

PTIOOSIN ☐☐☐☐☐☐☐☐ (12)

ECIAUOTDN ☐☐☐☐☐☐☐☐☐ (17)

KWEDNGOLE ☐☐☐☐☐☐☐☐☐

POSIASN ☐☐☐☐☐☐☐

☐☐☐☐ ☐☐☐☐ ☐☐☐☐☐☐☐

1 2 3 4   6 7 8 9   11 12 13 14 15 16 17

ISO Certification for SPD Departments & AAMI/ASTM Updates

https://directory.libsyn.com/episode/index/id/12117377

ISO Certification for SPD Departments

AAMI/ASTM Updates

M	A	O	P	E	R	A	T	I	O	N	R	T	T	S	Q
F	V	S	Q	N	T	J	S	C	I	L	A	N	O	E	A
D	N	T	Z	T	H	R	O	U	V	E	E	B	C	C	R
R	O	O	A	O	P	M	L	Y	A	M	C	X	T	N	S
A	G	C	M	S	P	T	T	R	T	A	E	F	N	M	T
T	J	K	U	A	W	I	S	R	D	M	I	B	E	J	S
I	X	O	R	M	L	C	A	T	Q	L	D	E	M	S	P
N	E	E	H	A	E	P	O	M	M	Y	Z	N	E	W	F
G	L	T	U	L	E	N	R	K	H	Y	A	C	V	W	Y
P	X	Q	A	D	O	H	T	E	M	F	O	H	O	T	C
E	H	A	B	D	O	L	X	F	G	R	L	M	R	G	U
G	Q	J	N	U	I	T	H	Z	P	B	X	A	P	Y	N
D	H	V	Y	O	K	L	N	M	W	C	E	R	M	E	K
C	Y	K	S	S	V	R	A	X	W	S	W	K	I	A	W
C	D	L	I	B	Q	R	C	V	O	C	B	R	P	E	W
S	E	R	A	C	H	T	L	A	E	H	N	C	A	L	N

VALIDATE
BENCHMARK
METHOD
COMPARE
DEPARTMENT
RISK
DOCUMENT
IMPROVEMENT
QUALITY
PROCESS
OPERATION
RATING
HEALTHCARE

ISO Certification for SPD Departments

AAMI/ASTM Updates

VIATALDE _ _ _ _ _ _ _ _ (6, 15)

ITRSCTUNONIS _ _ _ _ _ _ _ _ _ _ _ _ (1, 9)

MFRECNUAAUTR _ _ _ _ _ _ _ _ _ _ _ _ (12)

IKRS _ _ _ _

PEROSCS _ _ _ _ _ _ _

BMHNRACEK _ _ _ _ _ _ _ _ _ (17, 4)

DNMCEOUT _ _ _ _ _ _ _ _ (7, 14)

OAPOTREIN _ _ _ _ _ _ _ _ _ (5)

MTHOED _ _ _ _ _ _

IEVEMMPNROT _ _ _ _ _ _ _ _ _ _ _ (3, 10, 16)

RNIATG _ _ _ _ _ _

CARMPOE _ _ _ _ _ _ _ (2)

QLIATUY _ _ _ _ _ _ _

HAHRLEATCE _ _ _ _ _ _ _ _ _ _ (11)

DPTNEMEART _ _ _ _ _ _ _ _ _ _

_ _ _ _ _ _ _   _ _ _ _   _ _ _ _

1 2 3 4 5 6 7   9 10 11 12   14 15 16 17

A Winning Plan: Making Process Improvement Possible

https://directory.libsyn.com/episode/index/id/12623057

A Winning Plan

Making Process Improvement Possible

C	W	A	V	Q	A	M	E	A	S	U	R	A	B	L	E
I	T	N	O	M	W	Q	P	H	D	A	I	W	G	F	V
M	R	A	Y	S	K	K	P	R	R	Y	S	Z	Z	E	B
P	A	L	W	V	B	N	W	O	O	M	B	W	Y	T	G
R	I	Y	H	C	T	F	E	Y	E	J	O	V	N	Y	O
O	N	S	S	F	B	M	O	T	T	L	E	E	V	A	S
V	I	I	D	K	O	A	S	Q	F	P	T	C	P	E	T
E	N	S	W	C	F	Y	G	K	Y	S	K	S	T	Q	R
M	G	U	T	A	S	O	R	N	I	T	D	N	H	K	A
E	Q	U	N	O	S	O	T	S	M	V	A	N	K	E	C
N	O	C	I	O	W	T	N	V	K	L	C	V	F	M	K
T	K	F	R	F	S	O	E	W	P	K	R	A	C	J	I
U	N	T	O	H	C	L	D	Y	L	X	S	H	S	J	N
L	E	M	P	L	O	Y	E	E	J	Y	K	F	N	B	G
M	M	V	N	J	K	P	Y	O	K	M	A	F	F	U	X
O	J	P	O	Q	Q	B	M	L	I	M	R	K	J	C	T

EMPLOYEE
SYSTEM
WASTE
PLAN
WORKFLOW
SAFE
IMPROVEMENT
CONSISTENT
ANALYSIS
PROJECT
OUTCOME
TRAINING
SYSTEMS
TRACKING
MEASURABLE

A Winning Plan

Making Process Improvement Possible

EPYMEOLE
15

AESF

OOCMTUE
9 5 13

STYESM

IOVEPMRENMT
6 16

TIRIANNG

TWAES
3

CINESSONTT
11

SEMYSTS
1 8

ANLP

AILNSAYS

TAIRCNKG

WRFOLKOW

PJCEORT
14

MAUALSREBE
2 12

															D
1	2	3	5	6	8	9	11	12	13	14	15	16	17		

What Happened in Vegas: A Story About the Heart of Sterile Processing in the Midst of Tragedy

https://directory.libsyn.com/episode/index/id/12623078

What Happened in Vegas

The Heart of Sterile Processing in the Midst of Tragedy

Y	M	R	C	Y	Z	T	H	I	N	K	I	N	G	Z	G
P	W	O	Q	N	F	T	O	R	T	N	L	V	N	H	Z
D	Y	D	N	Z	U	R	B	T	C	U	Z	Q	F	P	S
E	E	R	R	R	H	A	P	L	A	N	N	I	N	G	C
F	S	R	E	B	I	U	L	Z	P	C	A	P	B	X	H
Y	F	S	A	T	Y	M	L	O	V	U	L	N	M	Y	E
G	F	J	E	P	S	A	I	Z	U	A	X	F	L	C	D
E	U	W	R	R	E	A	K	X	N	T	I	S	T	N	U
V	M	A	E	T	T	R	S	W	M	G	C	M	R	E	L
V	Y	C	S	A	T	S	P	I	O	Q	W	O	V	G	E
C	X	C	P	G	Y	H	C	C	D	I	Z	C	M	R	J
H	F	Y	O	D	X	B	R	B	P	C	E	B	A	E	T
M	B	V	N	V	A	I	I	W	F	M	F	I	H	M	F
P	Y	E	S	F	S	B	W	M	I	J	V	N	G	E	H
R	H	T	E	I	V	T	S	T	Z	V	H	M	V	C	G
Q	Y	B	S	A	M	X	F	W	N	V	Y	H	W	R	X

EMERGENCY
PLANNING
TRAUMA
SCHEDULE
THINKING
PREPARED
RESPONSE
TEAM
OUTCOME
PLAN
DISASTER
CRISIS
TIME
SKILL
STRESS

What Happened in Vegas

The Heart of Sterile Processing in the Midst of Tragedy

EEMCENRGY ☐☐☐☐☐☐☐☐☐ (6)

PAERPERD ☐☐☐☐☐☐☐☐ (7)

DTISSEAR ☐☐☐☐☐☐☐☐ (5)

PNNLNAIG ☐☐☐☐☐☐☐☐ (8, 15, 17)

ROENPSSE ☐☐☐☐☐☐☐☐

CIRISS ☐☐☐☐☐☐ (12)

TMRAUA ☐☐☐☐☐☐ (2)

ATME ☐☐☐☐

MEIT ☐☐☐☐ (4, 3)

SEUDLCHE ☐☐☐☐☐☐☐☐ (24, 1, 11, 23)

OTOUMCE ☐☐☐☐☐☐☐

ILLKS ☐☐☐☐☐ (19, 14)

TINKHNIG ☐☐☐☐☐☐☐☐ (21, 16, 20, 13)

NPLA ☐☐☐☐ (22)

SETSRS ☐☐☐☐☐☐ (10)

1 2 3 4 5 6 7 8   10 11 12 13 14 15 16 17   19 20 21 22 23 24

On Board for Improvement
Building Teams and Trust for a New Sterile Processing Leader

https://directory.libsyn.com/episode/index/id/12799856

On Board for Improvement

Building Teams and Trust for a New Sterile Processing Leader

W	D	E	N	R	A	V	I	M	X	X	G	M	E	J	T
C	Q	P	D	E	K	P	G	L	L	A	I	K	G	E	A
E	L	C	E	G	Y	S	S	W	L	R	R	W	L	T	C
L	P	S	N	R	K	G	H	S	E	Y	N	D	N	B	C
E	W	I	T	D	F	C	N	T	Q	T	D	E	M	I	O
B	A	E	N	R	H	O	N	E	S	U	M	X	K	O	U
R	S	W	A	P	A	I	R	U	H	E	O	U	Q	E	N
A	T	X	W	F	U	V	R	M	G	X	O	N	F	F	T
T	E	E	B	M	D	T	E	A	A	N	G	S	S	S	A
E	N	O	O	L	G	P	G	L	D	N	N	R	W	F	B
G	N	H	L	W	S	N	E	F	E	Z	C	Z	O	Z	I
Y	L	K	Z	B	E	A	Z	J	H	R	M	E	P	W	L
C	R	E	C	O	G	N	I	T	I	O	N	I	D	L	I
T	C	O	M	M	U	N	I	C	A	T	I	O	N	E	T
N	X	Q	I	U	A	V	H	A	M	S	X	F	R	A	Y
A	O	B	S	E	R	V	A	T	I	O	N	H	X	N	T

TRAVELER
INPUT
LEAN
ENGAGEMENT
RECOGNITION
TRUST
INTERIM
GROW
PERFORMANCE
ACCOUNTABILITY
COMMUNICATION
OBSERVATION
CELEBRATE
WASTE
HUDDLE

On Board for Improvement

Building Teams and Trust for a New Sterile Processing Leader

TELAREVR

10

ITRIENM

21

OOETVISBARN

NPTIU

13 5

OWRG

20

CLBERTEAE

14 2 18 19

ENLA

PCORNAEMFRE

8 7 17

TEASW

23

EMEEGANNGT

15 11

ALITOIBNUTCCAY

12 3

HDULDE

RNECOIOIGTN

6 22

CCAITMUNOMION

9

STTRU

K

1 2 3 5 6 7 8 9 10 11 12 13 14 15 17 18 19 20 21 22 23

Become a Triple-Threat Sterile Processing Leader

What Your Teams Need and Your Bosses Want

thought the day would never end. It was already three in the afternoon, and I'd been bouncing around from meeting to meeting all day, stealing precious moments in the hallway to coordinate final plans for the upcoming staff meeting by texting my manager.

"How do they expect us to get anything done around here?" I whispered to the OR Director, as I sat back down in the packed conference room. A knowing glance was all he gave in reply. As the presentation continued, I was fighting the urge to ignore the speaker and think about the other twenty things I needed to get done today so that tomorrow would go smoothly. "Zimmer," I scribbled on my notepad, trying to act like I was taking meeting notes. Actually, I wanted to remember that it's been three days since their case, and they still hadn't picked up their loaner trays from the outgoing loaner cart

There will be days in the life of every Sterile Processing professional when you feel like you've missed out on opportunities to really push your department forward. Whether you're a technician who planned to finally master that new Skull Base Instrument tray, a manager who had hoped to complete the PowerPoint for tomorrow's physician meeting, or a director who had ten emails to respond to, but also five fires to put out -- days have a way of escaping us without always giving us the satisfaction of checking off our to-do list.

The question is: what's the true priority? What does your team need from you in your current role and what should your boss expect? How you answer these questions has everything to do with how prepared you will be to dominate your next interview for a leadership role or how successful you'll be in your current position. You can distill the answer to these questions into three basic layers of effective Sterile Processing leadership, and in order to excel, you will need them all. Let's discuss them in order . . .

1. Technical

This first layer of leadership is the foundation for all the rest: technical know-how. There are no effective SPD leaders in the industry who do not understand the basic technical functions of their department. For front-line leaders such as team leads, supervisors, coordinators, and high-performing techs, this is the priority leadership function you should be providing to your team. Excelling here means becoming the department resource for instrument IFU questions, instrument tracking troubleshooting, care of reprocessing equipment/tools, department workflow, preference card interpretation, knowledge of both official and unofficial instrument storage locations, etc. There is a near endless supply of things to know, and at this level you should always be pushing yourself to know more. Be the sponge, and it won't be long until others treat you like a leader.

2. Relational

As you move up a level to supervisor and manager positions, the second layer of effective SPD leadership must take into account relational responsibilities. Take note that this next level is not supplanting technical know-how, it's merely building on top of it. This relational level is where many new department leaders are set up to fail. While they may have been the department experts in workflow, instrument knowledge, and documentation requirements, that does not mean they understand or can handle the relational side of higher-level leadership. Supervisors and managers deal with people just as much, if not more, than they deal with processes. So, to excel here you must intentionally cultivate strong relationships, both with your staff, among your staff, and with other department leaders. If you buy into the theory that 'they don't have to like me as long as they respect me,' you will fail. It's true, some people won't like you no matter what. But if no one likes you, it won't be long until you realize no one respects you either. Make it your priority to build strong relationships at this level and you'll be in a good position to move on to the next.

1. **Political**

The final aspect of this tri-level leadership model is political. Now, I know politics has become a dirty word in our day and age, but let's set that connotation aside for a moment and focus on what it means in our world. Once you step into a manager or director role in Sterile Processing, you become the de facto SPD expert in your facility. You'll be attending meetings with CNOs, COOs, OR Directors, and a host of other folks who have a general idea of what you do, but very little idea of how your team actually does it. This means your primarily responsibility at this level is to advocate for best practices, build coalitions with like-minded facility leaders, and set the broader agenda for your other department leaders. Unsurprisingly, for this political focus to be successful, it needs strong relationships (layer #2) and technical expertise (layer

#1). The CEO may not know how to run a sterilizer, but he usually knows when you don't know what you're talking about. When you need the OR Director's support in confronting a grumpy surgeon, you're gonna wish you wouldn't have strained your relationship by sending that snarky email to them last week. At this political level, you must be intentional about knowing how much cultural capital you have and knowing when to spend it -- for the good of your team.

To become an effective SPD leader, you must come to terms with these three levels of leadership, understand how they apply to where you are, and realize how they can take you to where you want to be. Some of the best front-line technicians I've ever known excelled because they knew how important relationships were to doing their jobs well. Some of the best supervisors and managers I've seen were intentional about reaching out to other department leaders and collaborating on mutually beneficial projects. Some of the most boring meetings I've ever been in have borne the greatest fruit because I was present to insist upon following industry best-practices.

Excellent SPD leadership cannot be one-dimensional. The only true danger to professional mediocrity is becoming a triple-threat Sterile Processing leader -- those who know the job, know their people, and know how to work within the system.

Here's to growth -- pressed down, shaken together, and running over.

W. Hank Balch ©

Every Second Matters: Frontline Insights and Perspectives from a 2nd Shift SPD Leader

https://directory.libsyn.com/episode/index/id/12799757

Every Second Matters

Frontline Insights and Perspectives from a 2nd Shift SPD Leader

B	R	O	S	I	V	R	E	P	U	S	H	L	D	V	C
I	I	Q	J	D	J	A	E	M	L	M	A	E	V	N	R
T	Z	C	J	S	J	S	R	D	O	O	V	T	O	Q	N
U	P	B	E	E	E	C	H	T	U	I	E	I	Z	O	X
B	E	W	F	N	L	Z	I	I	T	C	S	O	I	S	R
B	G	T	K	Q	G	V	S	C	F	S	A	T	F	E	I
P	X	B	B	J	A	A	A	R	A	T	A	T	O	H	K
E	O	V	R	T	P	O	G	P	A	R	V	W	I	S	G
E	Z	T	I	E	R	Z	X	I	I	W	S	P	S	O	B
Y	D	O	E	P	E	I	C	P	N	Q	U	G	S	Q	N
O	N	B	T	N	R	R	S	I	B	G	D	J	L	J	E
L	X	Q	C	C	T	N	A	E	C	I	O	V	O	I	I
P	R	D	Y	M	I	I	K	C	L	Y	L	X	N	D	B
M	X	R	K	W	I	Y	A	B	S	D	I	T	E	Q	F
E	B	Z	P	M	W	V	J	L	G	D	Y	A	S	G	A
E	D	U	T	I	T	T	A	J	P	H	S	U	N	B	U

SHIFT
EMPLOYEE
ENGAGING
VOICE
PASSION
SUPERVISOR
WARS
PROACTIVE
CAREER
INSPIRATION
MOTIVATION
EDUCATION
IDEAS
POTENTIAL
ATTITUDE

Every Second Matters

Frontline Insights and Perspectives from a 2nd Shift SPD Leader

Scrambled word	Boxes	Numbered boxes (box position → number)
HITSF	5	2 → 8; 5 → 4
SIEVUROPSR	10	2 → 11
MTOVOIAITN	10	
EEYOPMLE	8	4 → 15; 6 → 5; 8 → 19
SRWA	4	
EUCAIOTDN	9	2 → 18; 3 → 1; 7 → 23
ENGGINAG	8	1 → 16; 5 → 12
PCTOVIRAE	9	2 → 9
EADSI	5	
OICEV	5	
CEEARR	6	
PTTOEANIL	9	1 → 24; 2 → 10; 6 → 7
PIOASSN	7	2 → 17; 3 → 21
ISPOATRNIIN	11	2 → 2; 5 → 3; 6 → 20
AUTTIDTE	8	

1	2	3	4	5

7	8	9	10	11	12	13
						H

15	16	17	18	19	20	21	22	23	24
							H		

Dangers on the Orient(ation) Express: Getting On-boarding Right with Competency Based Programs

https://directory.libsyn.com/episode/index/id/12799865

Dangers on the Orient(ation) Express

Getting On-boarding Right with Competency Based Programs

M	D	E	V	E	L	O	P	M	E	N	T	O	L	S	E
L	E	A	R	N	I	N	G	W	K	O	N	F	E	C	O
C	U	C	P	X	C	O	M	P	B	T	N	C	H	J	R
O	N	O	I	E	Z	H	B	A	R	M	R	S	J	S	I
M	W	N	E	O	P	O	E	O	L	U	V	M	X	A	E
P	A	B	X	V	W	R	P	C	O	G	X	I	B	N	N
E	B	O	C	F	A	P	E	S	K	N	X	C	P	N	T
T	G	A	O	O	U	L	E	C	O	L	W	M	G	U	A
E	E	R	Q	S	L	R	I	I	E	P	I	N	V	A	T
N	Z	D	I	J	H	L	T	D	G	P	I	S	J	L	I
C	X	I	U	N	D	N	E	H	A	N	T	T	T	H	O
I	X	N	T	C	E	Z	S	G	I	T	F	O	O	X	N
E	B	G	Z	T	A	Z	Z	A	E	C	I	X	R	Q	N
S	I	P	E	G	T	T	R	Y	Z	B	A	O	V	Q	J
P	G	R	Z	I	M	T	O	U	G	I	A	O	N	T	N
A	H	K	O	W	K	F	E	R	A	Z	P	O	V	V	Q

COLLEGE	TRAINING	ORIENTATION
COMPETENCIES	ANNUAL	ONBOARDING
DEVELOPMENT	EDUCATOR	CHECKLIST
VALIDATION	PRECEPTOR	RETENTION
RESOURCES	LEARNING	SUPPORT

Dangers on the Orient(ation) Express

Getting On-boarding Right with Competency Based Programs

CLOEGLE [1] [10] [ ] [ ] [ ] [ ] [ ]

TNIRNIAG [ ] [11] [ ] [ ] [ ] [18] [ ] [ ]

OINAOITERTN [ ] [ ] [ ] [ ] [14] [15] [ ] [ ] [ ] [ ] [20]

CIPOTENCEEMS [ ] [19] [3] [ ] [ ] [ ] [ ] [ ] [ ] [ ] [13] [ ]

AUANNL [16] [ ] [ ] [ ] [ ] [5]

ODABINONRG [ ] [ ] [ ] [ ] [ ] [ ] [ ] [12] [ ] [ ]

DOEPMLNEVET [ ] [ ] [ ] [ ] [ ] [2] [4] [ ] [ ] [ ] [7]

EADOTCUR [ ] [ ] [ ] [ ] [ ] [ ] [ ] [ ]

CCLSIKHET [ ] [ ] [ ] [ ] [ ] [ ] [ ] [ ] [ ]

VIOLATIDAN [ ] [ ] [ ] [ ] [ ] [ ] [ ] [ ] [ ] [ ]

POPTCERER [ ] [ ] [6] [ ] [ ] [ ] [ ] [ ] [ ]

RENTOTEIN [ ] [8] [ ] [ ] [ ] [17] [ ] [ ] [ ]

RCESEORUS [ ] [ ] [ ] [ ] [ ] [ ] [ ] [ ] [ ]

LARNNEIG [ ] [ ] [ ] [ ] [ ] [ ] [ ] [ ]

SPRPUOT [ ] [ ] [ ] [ ] [ ] [ ] [ ]

[1] [2] [3] [4] [5] [6] [7] [8]   [10] [11] [12] [13] [14] [15] [16] [17] [18] [19] [20]

All Together Now: Sterile Processing Centralization

https://directory.libsyn.com/episode/index/id/15059375

All Together Now

Sterile Processing Centralization

S	T	E	R	I	L	I	Z	A	T	I	O	N	S	D	G
D	I	L	O	L	M	M	G	K	K	M	X	I	U	Y	W
W	T	F	S	P	J	O	M	V	O	W	B	J	P	F	C
H	P	D	R	V	R	N	S	K	N	E	R	B	P	O	W
H	Q	N	B	J	B	E	L	U	Y	K	J	G	L	T	E
K	T	X	H	Y	K	Y	F	A	R	R	J	X	Y	Q	C
W	C	S	E	R	V	I	C	E	Y	G	S	D	I	P	E
B	O	T	R	A	N	S	P	O	R	T	E	Y	O	S	N
I	D	R	S	S	G	K	U	N	D	E	T	O	C	X	T
E	P	H	K	N	O	I	H	Q	Q	I	N	I	N	E	R
M	Q	J	I	F	Z	B	I	X	L	V	T	C	Z	T	A
C	W	V	T	U	L	A	G	I	K	Y	Y	S	E	S	L
O	A	G	N	O	D	O	C	O	L	W	P	W	O	M	I
S	S	S	K	F	U	A	W	A	X	A	C	J	V	Y	Z
V	G	Y	S	A	F	R	N	S	N	I	L	X	X	Q	E
I	S	T	A	N	D	A	R	D	I	Z	E	M	W	Y	K

FACILITY
STANDARDIZE
SUPPLY
WORKFLOW
ANALYTICS
MONEY
SURGEON
STERILIZATION
SAVINGS
SERVICE
CENTRALIZE
PREFERENCE
TRANSPORT
TOUR

All Together Now

Sterile Processing Centralization

FIITACLY

EYMON
10

CLENZIRTAE
1 9

SDTZARNIDAE
3 11

SROEUGN
5 22

PRFECERENE
2

CITNMOCAUIMON
15 20 16 6

SLUPPY
13

SAOELITIZRITN
4 8

TONPRRSAT
14 21 19

WOFRLOKW
7

SIGNVAS
18

UROT

AYCTIALNS

SVICERE
17

1 2 3 4 5 6 7 8 9 10 11   13 14 15 16 17 18 19 20 21 22

The Goal is Zero:
An IUSS Success Story

https://directory.libsyn.com/episode/index/i
d/15059408

The Goal is Zero

An IUSS Success Story

N	S	T	E	R	I	L	I	Z	A	T	I	O	N	Q	L
M	N	K	H	P	Y	B	L	N	Q	N	F	K	M	K	X
E	M	S	V	T	P	P	X	V	V	L	G	C	I	B	F
N	H	D	D	L	Q	S	Y	S	T	E	M	O	H	I	F
O	I	B	I	N	S	T	R	U	M	E	N	T	I	O	M
F	L	L	N	M	Y	J	U	X	Z	T	S	T	V	B	I
M	S	U	U	I	O	Y	L	E	Y	E	N	J	O	U	N
R	O	U	E	W	M	R	P	O	L	I	C	Y	Z	R	G
V	Y	N	R	W	N	M	A	V	E	N	D	O	R	D	Y
P	O	I	I	G	P	C	E	L	E	B	X	F	Z	E	G
O	G	T	J	T	E	V	H	D	E	S	A	V	C	N	Y
N	G	R	Y	D	O	R	D	A	I	O	M	C	Y	Q	T
D	B	A	V	P	F	R	Y	F	N	A	E	H	K	D	C
G	C	Y	N	A	U	D	I	T	N	G	T	V	R	U	D
J	O	S	W	Q	D	S	R	N	K	O	E	E	H	T	P
G	R	T	Y	S	O	M	K	O	G	U	N	M	C	C	E

BIOBURDEN
AUDIT
INVENTORY
BACKUP
STERILIZATION
IMMEDIATE
CHANGE
POLICY
INSTRUMENT
TRAYS
VENDOR
MONITORING
SYSTEM
MORALE
SURGERY

The Goal is Zero

An IUSS Success Story

BBIUEDORN
13 14

IAEMTDIME
6

VNDOER

UDITA
2

CGNHAE

MIOTORNNIG

IVETRNNOY

PIOCLY
16 1

SSEYTM
15 18

BCUAKP

IENRNMSUTT
4

MRLOAE
9 8

SIAIZTTELOIRN
3 11

RSYTA
10

SRRUGEY
17

1 2 3 4 6 8 9 10 11 13 14 15 16 17 18

Reprocessing in the United Arab Emirates: A Story of Pandemic, Leadership & Innovation

https://directory.libsyn.com/episode/index/id/16171175

Reprocessing in the United Arab Emirates

A Story of Pandemic, Leadership & Innovation

Q	K	G	E	I	U	G	J	S	K	S	A	M	V	J	A
K	E	V	I	T	C	A	O	R	P	H	D	H	B	E	J
T	N	O	I	T	A	D	N	U	O	F	R	D	Y	Q	Y
J	K	B	G	C	I	M	E	D	N	A	P	U	A	U	E
I	L	S	E	V	X	N	O	N	B	E	I	I	Q	I	Z
N	G	S	K	G	U	K	L	E	V	A	R	T	T	P	D
C	F	M	G	R	E	T	A	D	I	D	N	A	C	M	N
N	E	Z	S	R	H	K	E	C	S	W	Q	Z	U	E	U
E	G	I	J	G	I	J	O	A	A	X	C	V	S	N	O
C	N	F	N	O	S	U	Y	W	D	A	C	U	N	T	R
G	I	I	Z	W	N	Z	U	K	S	E	G	V	C	U	G
L	N	D	M	T	Y	U	S	E	V	U	G	J	I	W	K
A	I	C	R	B	W	I	S	H	M	I	S	R	S	G	C
J	A	Y	C	I	P	G	L	B	E	M	T	E	E	M	A
P	R	J	P	U	C	L	A	T	I	P	S	O	H	E	B
C	T	A	N	R	K	K	Q	J	R	V	V	K	E	J	F

COUNTRY
NURSING
FOUNDATION
EQUIPMENT
CASES
HOSPITAL
BACKGROUND
TRAINING
TRAVEL
PROACTIVE
CANDIDATE
DEGREE
PANDEMIC
MASKS

Reprocessing in the United Arab Emirates

A Story of Pandemic, Leadership & Innovation

CRTONUY — 7

HSTIAPOL — 8, 10

DCOIEANOAMNITTN — 12, 4, 23, 22, 17

CTDAANIDE — 5, 24

NISUNRG — 6

BNKACGROUD — 14, 15

DEEGRE

FTOIANUODN — 18

TINNIARG — 1, 11, 19

PMDEAINC — 2

EPMQNIUET — 20, 16

TEVRAL

KSMAS — 3

SSEAC

PIRCVOATE — 21

1 2 3 4 5 6 7 8   10 11 12   14 15 16 17 18 19 20 21 22 23 24

You're Gonna Miss Me When I'm Gone:

How Incomplete Surgical Trays Kill Your Culture and What You Can Do to Get It Back

A little over two years ago, one of my facilities had a missing instrument list of nearly two thousand instruments.

This meant that on a daily basis, we had two thousand culture-killers roaming around the OR, eating away at any hope we had at giving excellent customer service to our surgical services team -- physicians, nurses, techs -- and ultimately prohibiting us from giving the best possible care to our patients.

Surgical instrument trays can range in size anywhere from a single instrument up to over a hundred, each with its own particular combination of clamps, scissors, forceps, or needle holders. But when any one of those items is missing from a sterile instrument tray, it signals to the OR team that our production process is broken.

Overcoming this negative cultural pressure is the burden of nearly every Sterile Processing leader in the country. If you want to regain the culture of excellence laid out for your SPD team, you have to find a way to neutralize the damage done by incomplete surgical trays, and you need to do it quickly. Here are a few ideas that could help turn the cultural tide...

1. Tech Yourself Before You Wreck Yourself

A Sterile Processing technician is only as good as the tools they have to do their job. In terms of tackling a missing instrument list, you will need the best data possible located in all possible places. If you do not utilize an instrument tracking system and

don't have the capital to purchase one, comb through your paper count sheets to ensure every listing is as up-to-date as it can be (including cross-referenced instrument catalog numbers). If you are already computerized, you can do the same, only quicker -- hopefully. This is one of the most labor-intensive parts of driving down a huge missing list, but it's the only way to ensure your technicians can trust the count sheet in front of them as they process each tray. If "completing" a tray is a guessing game or a memory challenge for your department, errors will slide through, and your quality will inevitably take two steps back.

2. Ain't No Mountain High Enough

Although the numbers may start out at an overwhelming level, you can overcome them with the right amount of teamwork between your department and the OR. I would recommend you start with the low hanging fruit of instrument sets missing instruments that are rarely used. Approach your service line leaders or OR coordinators about removing the tray from inventory completely or at least deleting instruments that have viable substitutes in other trays. Use the large number of total missing instruments to your advantage (at the beginning) and highlight how negative of an impact this can have on patient safety and processing efficiencies. Share it with everyone who will listen -- vendors, physicians, facility leadership, and OR staff. The more widespread the knowledge is of your current state, the larger the celebration will be when you finally tackle it.

3. If They Can Find It, They Will Come

Few things are more frustrating for front line techs than to be processing along at full speed, noticing an instrument is missing, and then knowing it will take them forever to find the proper replacement. Whether you utilize a drawer system, peg board, or bin storage for your backup instrumentation -- the key to success here is organization. Personally, I'm a fan of bin storage because it allows you to see the instruments (unlike the drawer system) and removing an instrument is not as difficult as with a crowded peg board (plus you can really make a bin system look sharp if you want to). The cultural impact of an organized backup inventory can mean the difference between a tech who happily spends 20 seconds finding the exact needle holder they need and a tech who begrudgingly leaves their table for a 10-minute excursion to the graveyard of productivity, a.k.a. the rat's nest of a backup wall you have. Don't make your techs choose between a productive night and completed surgical trays. They should want and be able to do both.

As we all know, decontamination is not the optimum processing location to be counting instruments and comparing against a tray profile, so the soonest most of us will be able to identify these issues will be in the prep/pack stage. Finding a streamlined way of determining where the tray was last used and collating that data in an easily readable format is something that could really solve a process issue that countless departments around the country struggle with (*take note all you instrument tracking software designers out there!*).

4. Let the Numbers and the Money Talk

As they say in the HR world, "If you didn't document it, it didn't happen." The same is true for instrumentation that doesn't make it back from the OR in our surgical trays. Without immediate/proper documentation of items that take a one-way trip to the surgical suite, it becomes very difficult to impact the culture that allows instruments to go AWOL in the first place.

But either way, the one sure place this information will show up is on your monthly instrument replacement budget. Take this number to every leadership meeting you attend, and let the money tell the story.

Ultimately, large numbers of missing instruments in your inventory are just as much a cultural issue as they are a process issue. Find your OR advocates (often the frustrated surgeon or OCD scrub tech) who understand the importance of what you're trying to do for the good of patient care and leverage that support to effect change in the OR. In your own department, give your team the tools they need to quickly and consistently process complete trays and find ways to gather the documentation you need to tell the story, both of the current cultural challenges and your eventual victory over them.

The only thing missing now is news of your success.

Go get 'em, cowboy.

W. Hank Balch ©

Solutions

Industry Certifications, Research Studies - Solution

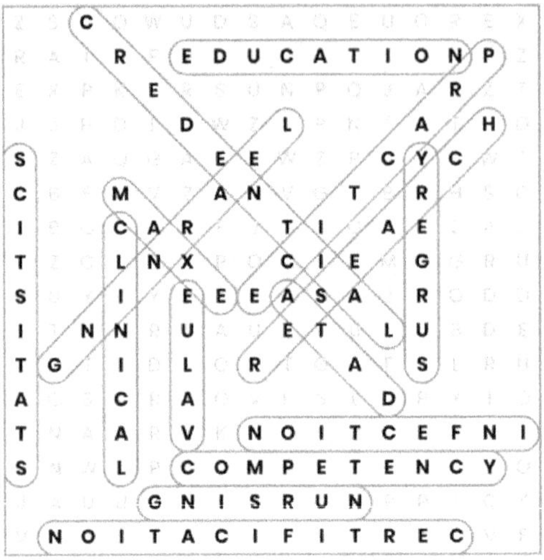

The Power of Data - Solution

Industry Certifications, Research Studies on Certification Impact

CRAIETCOFITIN	CERTIFICATION	T (4), O (20)
PCRIACTE	PRACTICE	P (8), C (19)
AEMX	EXAM	M (21)
CERNATEDIL	CREDENTIAL	E (5)
NRNIUSG	NURSING	
CINICALL	CLINICAL	I (11)
CPENEOCMTY	COMPETENCY	T (18), E (22)
IFIOENCTN	INFECTION	E (2), O (16), N (13)
AADT	DATA	
UVELA	VALUE	
SGERURY	SURGERY	U (17), R (6)
ECAITOUDN	EDUCATION	E (12)
RECASERH	RESEARCH	A (9)
LNRIENAG	LEARNING	
STISITACTS	STATISTICS	S (23), T (3), T (10), T (14)

BETTER PATIENT OUTCOMES

The CS Professional as a Patient - Solution

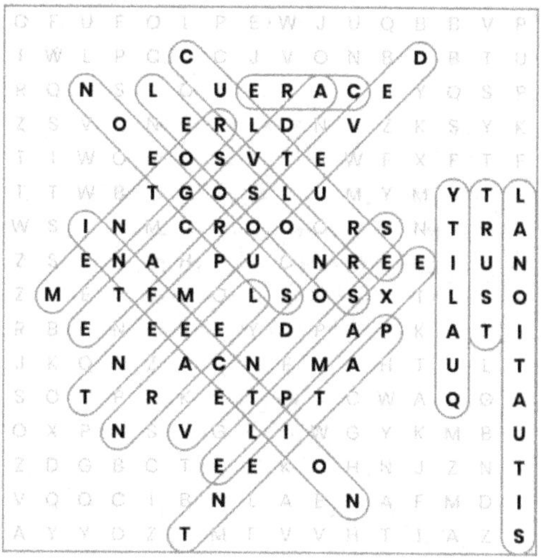

The CS Professional as a Patient - Solution

Lessons in Leadership and Surgical Instrument Quality

PINETAT	PATIENT	P 21, A 14, I 20
UTTRS	TRUST	S 3
CRULUTE	CULTURE	
QTIAULY	QUALITY	
SEGUORN	SURGEON	S 7, E 16
IINCTFOEN	INFECTION	I 9
VNDREOS	VENDORS	N 6
LSOSNES	LESSONS	L 12, S 18, O 5, N 10, S 4
ANREL	LEARN	R 17
MNTOER	MENTOR	
DLPEMVNEOET	DEVELOPMENT	D 15, E 13, L 1
EPMXLAE	EXAMPLE	E 2
AOTVDCAE	ADVOCATE	

LESSONS IN LEADERSHIP

Business Training for SPD Leaders - Solution

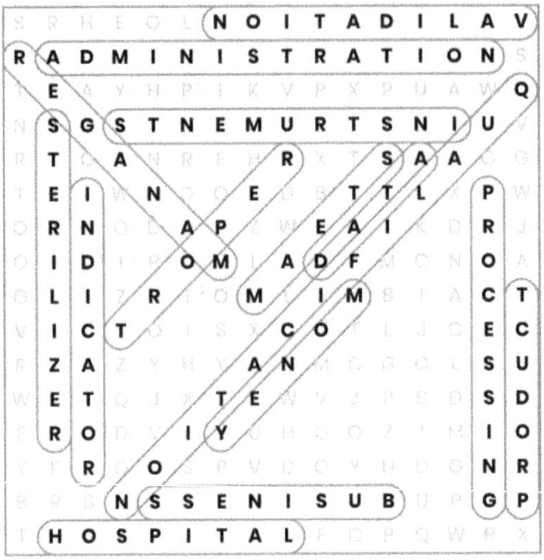

Business Training for SPD Leaders - Solution

Thermal Validation

MAEGNAR	MANAGER	M = 1, N = 3, G = 5
YEMNO	MONEY	Y = 14
POCRDUT	PRODUCT	P = 20
SIIETRZLER	STERILIZER	I = 6
ESMTA	STEAM	E = 13
ITRNUNTSMES	INSTRUMENTS	N = 17, N = 7
PISRSCONEG	PROCESSING	O = 11, G = 8
HIPTSAOL	HOSPITAL	S = 19
VLADITOAIN	VALIDATION	A = 2
ATDA	DATA	D = 21, A = 4
IINCTDOAR	INDICATOR	I = 16
BESUSNIS	BUSINESS	
RREPOT	REPORT	
AMNOITITASRIDN	ADMINISTRATION	M = 10, N = 12
QFUICIOTLAIAN	QUALIFICATION	

MANAGING MONEY IN SPD

OR/SPD Collaboration - Solution

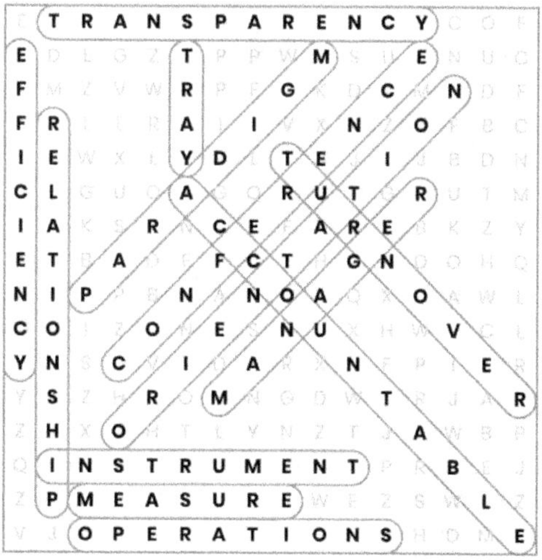

OR/SPD Collaboration - Solution

The OR Today Live Conference

CALROAOTIBOLN	COLLABORATION	C 6, L 8, A 10, B 11, N 18
PGAHARICNMAGDE	PARADIGMCHANGE	
CRNENECOFE	CONFERENCE	O 7, E 2
MRSUEAE	MEASURE	M 4
OIOAPRENTS	OPERATIONS	O 17, I 16
EFCIINCEFY	EFFICIENCY	
ACNBOAUTLCE	ACCOUNTABLE	A 14, O 12
TRSNNCAAPERY	TRANSPARENCY	A 3
ATYR	TRAY	T 1, R 13
RHOLINSEITAP	RELATIONSHIP	L 9
MAEGNAR	MANAGER	
IETRNSNUMT	INSTRUMENT	
TEUOVRNR	TURNOVER	
ONOITARETIN	ORIENTATION	T 15

TEAM COLLABORATION

Discovering Your Why - Solution

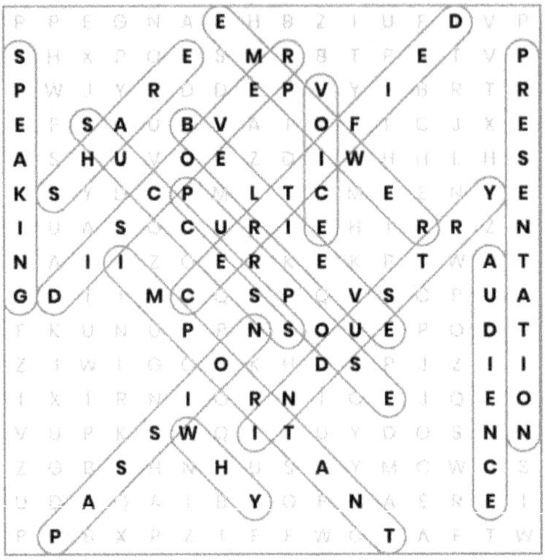

Discovering Your Why - Solution

Finding Your Voice and Public Speaking

CETIRIEFD	C E R T I F I E D	19 (F)
HYW	W H Y	12 (Y)
DOIVESCR	D I S C O V E R	15 (R)
SIPKENAG	S P E A K I N G	
PTNOIAERTSEN	P R E S E N T A T I O N	2 (E), 16 (S), 10 (N)
POIASSN	P A S S I O N	9 (I)
ICOEV	V O I C E	6 (V), 13 (O)
POPUSRE	P U R P O S E	
IUTRNSDY	I N D U S T R Y	
ADICUENE	A U D I E N C E	14 (U), 4 (I), 7 (E)
HERSA	S H A R E	17 (E)
BVIEELE	B E L I E V E	1 (B), 3 (L)
ITARPNMOT	I M P O R T A N T	
EOEPMWR	E M P O W E R	
SCESUCS	S U C C E S S	5 (E)

B E L I E V E   I N   Y O U R S E L F

An Industry in Transition - Solution

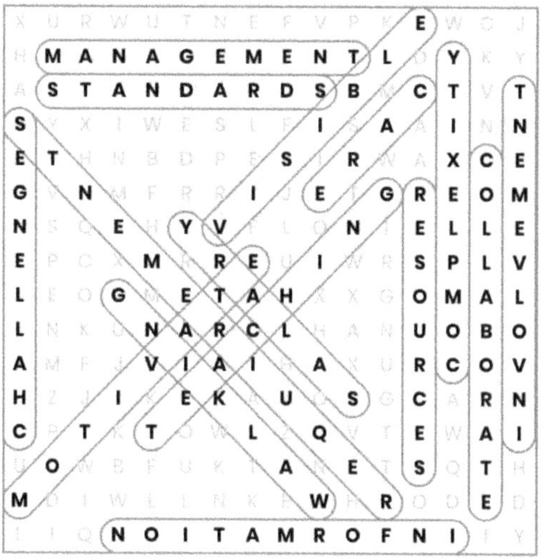

An Industry in Transition - Solution

Stories from the Trenches

CLIEPMOTXY	COMPLEXITY	Y (7)
RNTQEEEIMURS	REQUIREMENTS	U (20), R (18)
IMNFOARIOTN	INFORMATION	
RCUREESOS	RESOURCES	O (19)
WINALKG	WALKING	W (9), A (10), K (12)
TINECAHG	TEACHING	A (3)
ECAR	CARE	
MAOTTIVE	MOTIVATE	I (13)
VLIBISE	VISIBLE	B (6), E (2)
CLOORTABALE	COLLABORATE	L (1)
CANGHELELS	CHALLENGES	G (15)
SRAALY	SALARY	
IVLMNOVENET	INVOLVEMENT	N (14), L (11)
MNEAMNEGAT	MANAGEMENT	A (17), N (21)
SDATARDNS	STANDARDS	D (4), D (22)

LEAD BY WALKING AROUND

Sterile Processing Certification - Solution

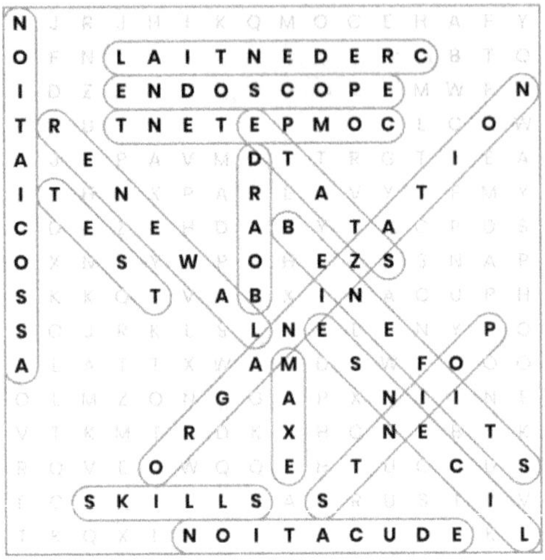

Sterile Processing Certification - Solution

The CBSPD Spotlight

Scrambled	Solution	Numbered letters
MEXA	EXAM	
EUADOICTN	EDUCATION	D 13, U 2, A 18, I 7
ATTES	STATE	
ADROB	BOARD	B 19, A 3
OTIIROAGAZNN	ORGANIZATION	N 12, A 16
LESNCIE	LICENSE	C 15
ACTIOISAOSN	ASSOCIATION	A 11
ESTT	TEST	
SILKLS	SKILLS	L 4, L 20
EOCDNPOSE	ENDOSCOPE	E 21, D 9
REANEWL	RENEWAL	
PNOTIS	POINTS	P 17
CENMTEPOT	COMPETENT	
CIETAERNDL	CREDENTIAL	E 8, I 5
BNIEETFS	BENEFITS	F 6

QUALIFIED AND CAPABLE

Surveying the Surveyor - Solution

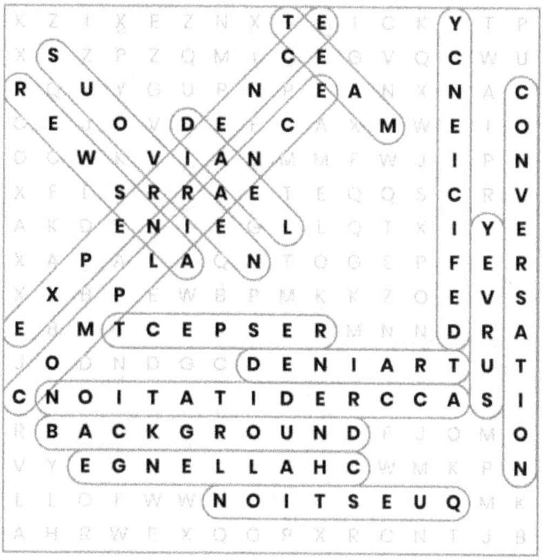

Surveying the Surveyor - Solution

What You Need to Know

Scrambled	Answer	Numbered letters
SEVURY	SURVEY	S (3)
BOGUKCRNAD	BACKGROUND	
QOUISETN	QUESTION	Q (12), U (13), I (17), O (18)
AWESNR	ANSWER	N (2), W (4), E (14)
ENIPEXRCEE	EXPERIENCE	
DCEEFCIINY	DEFICIENCY	
AOIAIRECCTDTN	ACCREDITATION	T (16)
TNEAIRD	TRAINED	R (6), A (1)
MTEA	TEAM	E (5)
CAPONCIMLE	COMPLIANCE	N (19)
NUOEVRS	NERVOUS	
ADEL	LEAD	
CSORNOAVIETN	CONVERSATION	T (8)
CLNELAGHE	CHALLENGE	H (9)
RCEESPT	RESPECT	S (15), E (10)

ANSWER THE QUESTION

Expertise vs Accreditation - Solution

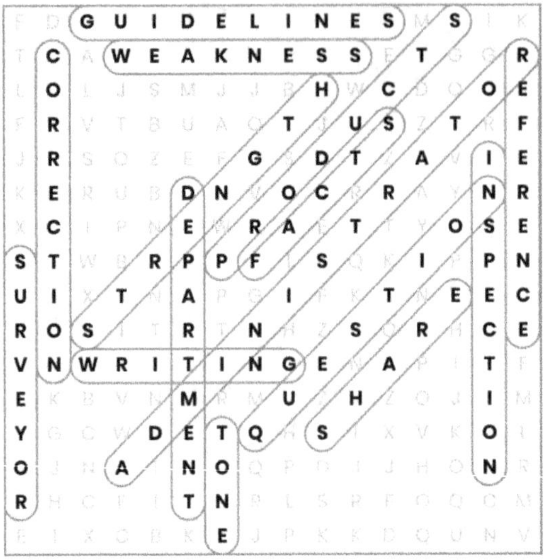

Expertise vs Accreditation - Solution

Challenges to the Surveying Process

STTGRNEH	STRENGTH	S (1), E (12), H (11)
WASEEKNS	WEAKNESS	K (5), S (18)
TCFSA	FACTS	F (14), C (4)
GDNEEIIULS	GUIDELINES	
CRITOOCREN	CORRECTION	C (16), T (2)
WITNRIG	WRITING	
QEOIUTSN	QUESTION	T (17)
REECNREFE	REFERENCE	
AOTAMDNISIRTR	ADMINISTRATOR	T (7)
IICONPESTN	INSPECTION	I (3), O (8)
PUTODRCS	PRODUCTS	
DNRMTEPAET	DEPARTMENT	A (15)
SVORUEYR	SURVEYOR	
ESHAR	SHARE	
ENTO	TONE	T (10)

STICK TO THE FACTS

The $50 Billion Dollar Opportunity - Solution

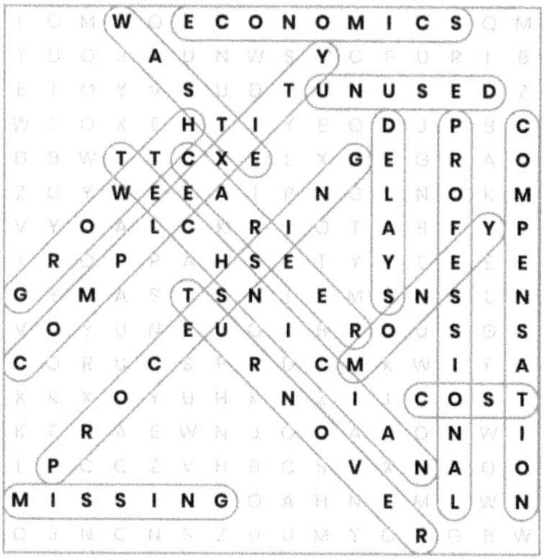

The $50 Billion Dollar Opportunity - Solution

Re-Thinking the Economics of Sterile Processing

TWESA	WASTE	A = 10
TRVOENUR	TURNOVER	U = 4, R = 16, O = 18, V = 19, R = 21
PERNSCSOIG	PROCESSING	S = 8
USNEUD	UNUSED	U = 15, D = 3
OTCS	COST	T = 14
CPNMTOEOASIN	COMPENSATION	
CLXOEMITPY	COMPLEXITY	T = 9
DLAYES	DELAYS	
MNISSIG	MISSING	
CEEARR	CAREER	R = 1, E = 20
GTROWH	GROWTH	
ENMOICCOS	ECONOMICS	E = 2, N = 17
NMYOE	MONEY	
THIICNACEN	TECHNICIAN	C = 5
PAINSOERSOFL	PROFESSIONAL	F = 11, E = 6

REDUCE STAFF TURNOVER

High Marks & High Standards - Solution

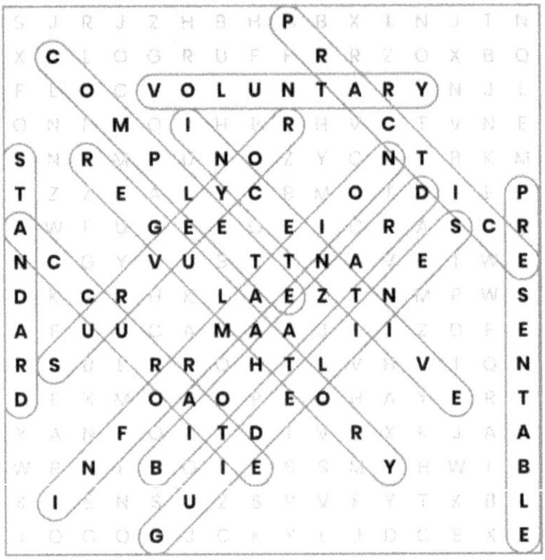

High Marks & High Standards - Solution

Compliant Reprocessing of Reusable Medical Devices

SANRTDAD	STANDARD	
GEDLUNIEIS	GUIDELINES	E (6), S (7)
RIEDOCAMNTOEMN	RECOMMENDATION	D (3)
IVINCETNE	INCENTIVE	
PCIARCTE	PRACTICE	P (10), T (8), I (15)
IRMAFOINTON	INFORMATION	
SVORUEYR	SURVEYOR	S (1), E (17)
VROAUNLTY	VOLUNTARY	
CPOEMTLE	COMPLETE	P (2)
AUATCRCE	ACCURATE	C (13)
PSANBELETRE	PRESENTABLE	T (14), B (5)
ADAIIOTCRETCN	ACCREDITATION	A (12), C (16)
RTOGARULEY	REGULATORY	R (11)
BRAAIHOZD	BIOHAZARD	
DONIEIANMATTCON	DECONTAMINATION	

S P D B E S T P R A C T I C E

Policies & Patients - Solution

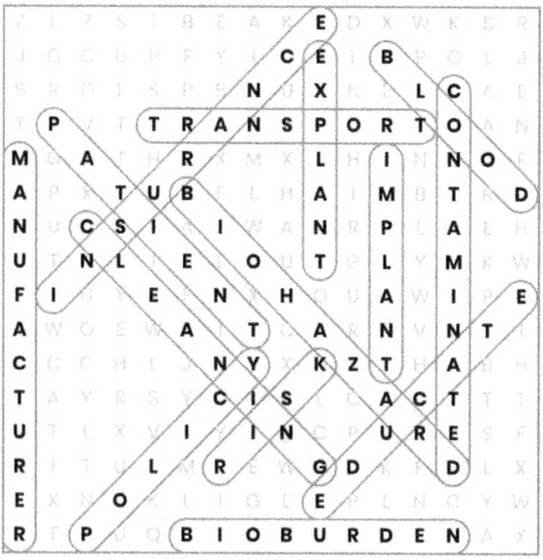

Policies & Patients - Solution

Insights on Explant Reprocessing

ILANMPT	I M P L A N T
EAXPNLT	E X[15] P[16] L A N T
PNIATET	P A T I E N T
MEUCTFAUANRR	M A N U F A C T U R E[2] R
CAAONNMTTEID	C O[5] N T A M I N A T[20] E D
BAZRHIAOD	B I O H A Z A[18] R D
IRACUNSNE	I N[19] S[9] U R[1] A N[11] C E
CNLNIEAG	C L[17] E[7] A N I N G[12]
PLICOY	P[3] O L I C[6] Y
ECDATUE	E D U C A T E[14]
TONPARSRT	T R A N S[21] P O R[4] T
ITNISTNUORCS	I N S[8] T R U C T I O N S
DOOBL	B L O O D
BUIEDOBRN	B I[10] O B U R D E N
KRIS	R I S K

R E P R O C E S S I N G E X P L A N T S

Higher Education - Solution

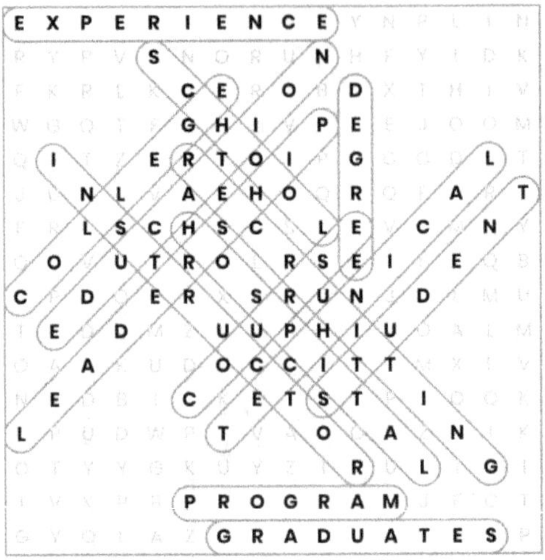

Higher Education - Solution

Collaborating With Technical Colleges

EAIDTOCUN	EDUCATION	C 12, O 20
SOCOHL	SCHOOL	H 4
TCHACEINL	TECHNICAL	C 3, A 23
RIINRECUTG	RECRUITING	G 21
HTOISAPL	HOSPITAL	O 14, I 6, A 8, L 9
LERADIESHP	LEADERSHIP	E 2, H 13
GUREADATS	GRADUATES	T 1
DGREEE	DEGREE	R 22
ITUCTNROSR	INSTRUCTOR	R 19, C 7, O 15
EEXPICRENE	EXPERIENCE	P 18
SDNUTET	STUDENT	S 11, N 5
IPRMEOMENVT	IMPROVEMENT	M 24
CLEOGLE	COLLEGE	L 16
CRSUOE	COURSE	

TECHNICAL SCHOOL PROGRAM

Certified Quality - Solution

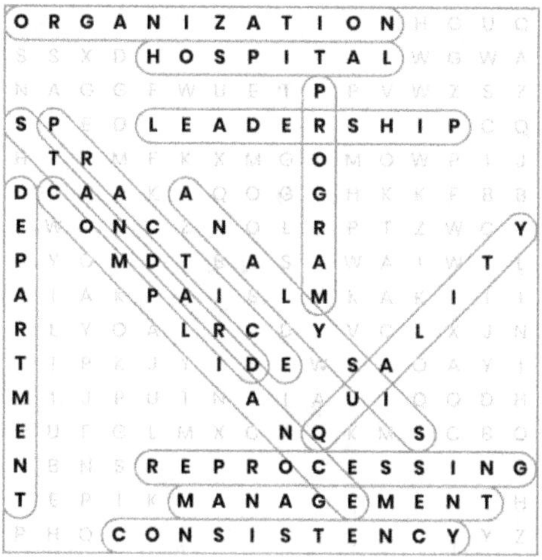

Certified Quality - Solution

Taking Sterile Processing Surveys to the Next Level

QLIATUY	Q U A L I T Y	A 4, T 21
MNAENEGMAT	M A N A G E M E N T	N 9, E 13
SAARTNDD	S T A N D A R D	
CCSONINTSEY	C O N S I S T E N C Y	C 19, T 10
CIECFATOIITRN	C E R T I F I C A T I O N	F 17, I 18, T 6
HIOSTAPL	H O S P I T A L	O 23, P 3
AYIALNSS	A N A L Y S I S	N 24
ARODCACIIETTN	A C C R E D I T A T I O N	R 5, E 8, D 1, I 22
RESNEPCRISOG	R E P R O C E S S I N G	C 12, E 2
LAEISEHDRP	L E A D E R S H I P	R 14
CALICMNPOE	C O M P L I A N C E	M 7
DNATEMEPRT	D E P A R T M E N T	T 15
PAGRORM	P R O G R A M	
OGTAIRAOZINN	O R G A N I Z A T I O N	I 16
PCITACRE	P R A C T I C E	A 20

D E P A R T M E N T   C E R T I F I C A T I O N

Insights from South Africa - Solution

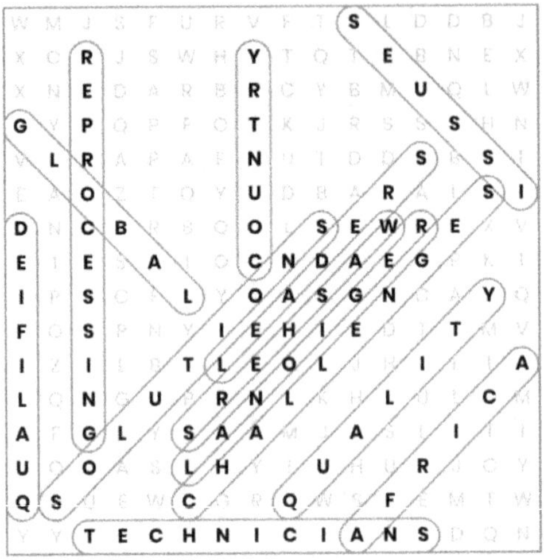

Insights from South Africa - Solution

Sterile Processing Perspectives and Regional Challenges

ARCFIA	AFRICA	I 9, A 7
PVEICSRETEPS	PERSPECTIVES	
RNEGIAOL	REGIONAL	G 19, I 18, N 2
CEEGNLHALS	CHALLENGES	H 20, N 16, S 22
QAIIELFUD	QUALIFIED	
CNSOAIOMEPTN	COMPENSATION	N 6, A 12, T 3, N 11
QAIUTLY	QUALITY	T 21
CUTORNY	COUNTRY	T 8
SNTOUOILS	SOLUTIONS	O 10
ISUESS	ISSUES	
TCCNIENHIAS	TECHNICIANS	I 1, I 15
LAREEDS	LEADERS	L 13, E 4
GBAOLL	GLOBAL	
RPRSESNECOIG	REPROCESSING	R 5
WHERASS	WASHERS	S 17

INTERNATIONAL INSIGHTS

The Good, the Bad, and the Ugly - Solution

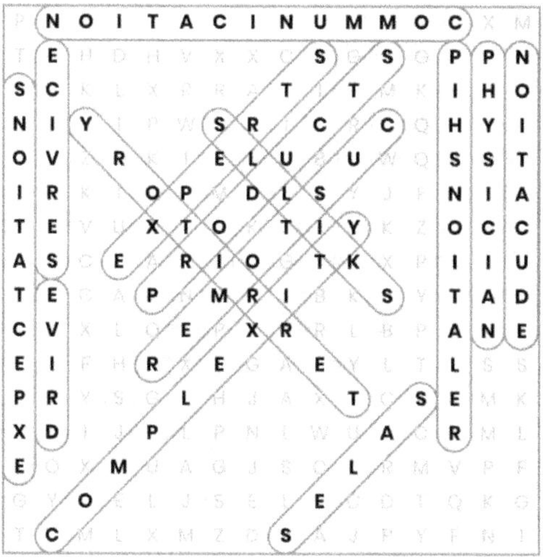

The Good, the Bad, and the Ugly - Solution

What to Look For In a Medical Device Sales Representative

REATETNRPSVEIE	REPRESENTATIVE	E 13, S 14, T 20
SCEIRVE	SERVICE	S 19, E 7
PUROCTDS	PRODUCTS	U 2
LEASS	SALES	
TTRREORIY	TERRITORY	O 5, R 18
EREXTPS	EXPERTS	
EODATUCIN	EDUCATION	O 11
SLKILS	SKILLS	
CUICTOAIOMNMN	COMMUNICATION	C 1, M 12, C 10
COMSTEUR	CUSTOMER	S 3, M 6, R 8
RTAISNELIOHP	RELATIONSHIP	T 4
PICAYISHN	PHYSICIAN	I 17
EIVDR	DRIVE	
CTPIMXLOEY	COMPLEXITY	
EETPINXAOTCS	EXPECTATIONS	

CUSTOMER COMES FIRST

The Human Connection - Solution

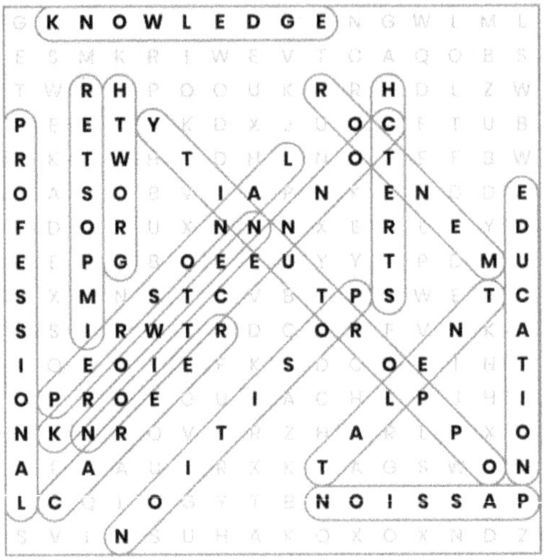

The Human Connection - Solution

Networking and Success in Sterile Processing

MNTOER	MENTOR	O = 2
CTOCNNIOEN	CONNECTION	
ONPPTIRUTOY	OPPORTUNITY	U = 3, Y = 1
CEERAR	CAREER	
TENLAT	TALENT	
PAOSFSIONREL	PROFESSIONAL	P = 6, F = 11, A = 15
PSENAORL	PERSONAL	R = 16, A = 7
GOWTRH	GROWTH	R = 4, T = 8, H = 9
ITSEMOPR	IMPOSTER	R = 13
NTREWOK	NETWORK	W = 14
SCTRTEH	STRETCH	
PTIOOSIN	POSITION	O = 12
ECIAUOTDN	EDUCATION	D = 17
KWEDNGOLE	KNOWLEDGE	
POSIASN	PASSION	

YOUR PATH FORWARD

ISO Certification for SPD Departments - Solution

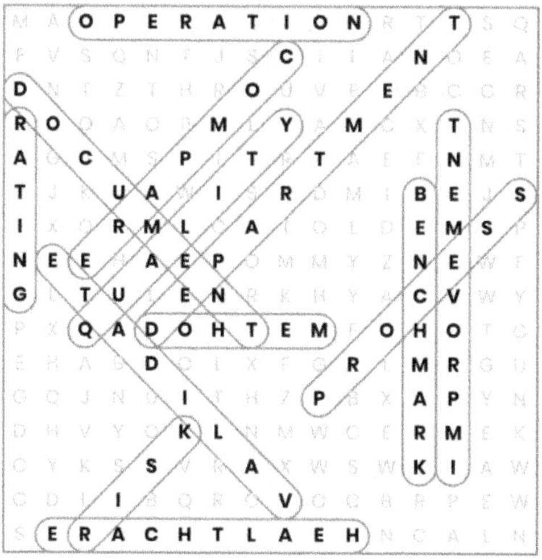

ISO Certification for SPD Departments - Solution

AAMI/ASTM Updates

VIATALDE	VALIDATE	V 6, I 15
ITRSCTUNONIS	INSTRUCTIONS	I 1, O 9
MFRECNUAAUTR	MANUFACTURER	R 12
IKRS	RISK	
PEROSCS	PROCESS	
BMHNRACEK	BENCHMARK	E 17, R 4
DNMCEOUT	DOCUMENT	E 7, T 14
OAPOTREIN	OPERATION	O 5
MTHOED	METHOD	
IEVEMMPNROT	IMPROVEMENT	P 3, V 10, M 16
RNIATG	RATING	
CARMPOE	COMPARE	M 2
QLIATUY	QUALITY	
HAHRLEATCE	HEALTHCARE	E 11
DPTNEMEART	DEPARTMENT	

IMPROVE OVER TIME

A Winning Plan - Solution

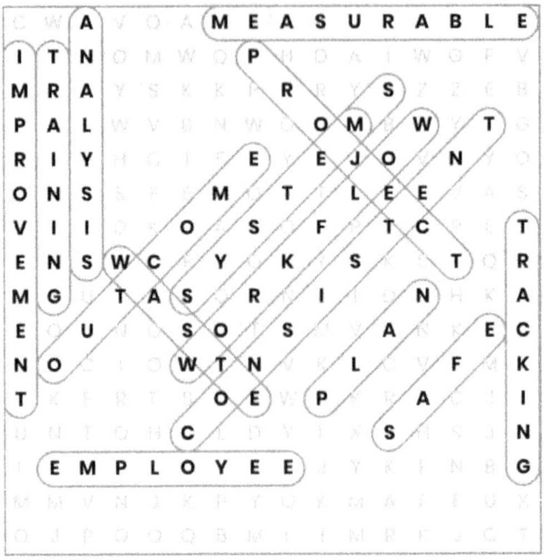

A Winning Plan - Solution

Making Process Improvement Possible

Scrambled	Answer	Numbered letters
EPYMEOLE	EMPLOYEE	E (15)
AESF	SAFE	
OOCMTUE	OUTCOME	O (9), U (5), C (13)
STYESM	SYSTEM	
IOVEPMRENMT	IMPROVEMENT	P (6), E (16)
TIRIANNG	TRAINING	
TWAES	WASTE	T (3)
CINESSONTT	CONSISTENT	S (11)
SEMYSTS	SYSTEMS	S (1), T (8)
ANLP	PLAN	
AILNSAYS	ANALYSIS	
TAIRCNKG	TRACKING	
WRFOLKOW	WORKFLOW	
PJCEORT	PROJECT	C (14)
MAUALSREBE	MEASURABLE	E (2), U (12)

SET UP TO SUCCEED

What Happened in Vegas - Solution

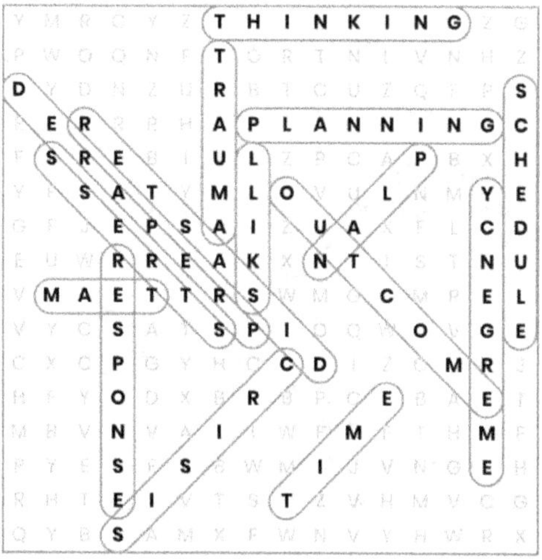

What Happened in Vegas - Solution

The Heart of Sterile Processing in the Midst of Tragedy

EEMCENRGY	E M E R G E N C Y	C = 6
PAERPERD	P R E P A R E D	A = 7
DTISSEAR	D I S A S T E R	I = 5
PNNLNAIG	P L A N N I N G	L = 8, I = 15, G = 17
ROENPSSE	R E S P O N S E	
CIRISS	C R I S I S	I = 12
TMRAUA	T R A U M A	R = 2
ATME	T E A M	
MEIT	T I M E	T = 4, I = 3
SEUDLCHE	S C H E D U L E	S = 24, C = 1, H = 11, L = 23
OTOUMCE	O U T C O M E	
ILLKS	S K I L L	S = 19, K = 14
TINKHNIG	T H I N K I N G	I = 21, N = 16, K = 20, N = 13
NPLA	P L A N	L = 22
SETSRS	S T R E S S	T = 10

C R I T I C A L T H I N K I N G S K I L L S

On Board for Improvement - Solution

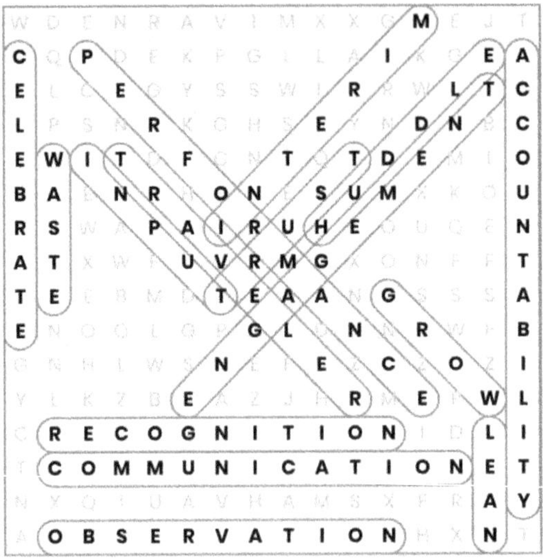

On Board for Improvement - Solution

Building Teams and Trust for a New Sterile Processing Leader

Scrambled	Answer	Numbered letters
TELAREVR	TRAVELER	R (10)
ITRIENM	INTERIM	I (21)
OOETVISBARN	OBSERVATION	
NPTIU	INPUT	N (13), P (5)
OWRG	GROW	R (20)
CLBERTEAE	CELEBRATE	C (14), E (2), E (18), T (19)
ENLA	LEAN	
PCORNAEMFRE	PERFORMANCE	F (8), R (7), M (17)
TEASW	WASTE	S (23)
EMEEGANNGT	ENGAGEMENT	E (15), M (11)
ALITOIBNUTCCAY	ACCOUNTABILITY	A (12), Y (3)
HDULDE	HUDDLE	
RNECOIOIGTN	RECOGNITION	E (6), C (22)
CCAITMUNOMION	COMMUNICATION	O (9)
STTRU	TRUST	

KEY PERFORMANCE METRICS

Every Second Matters - Solution

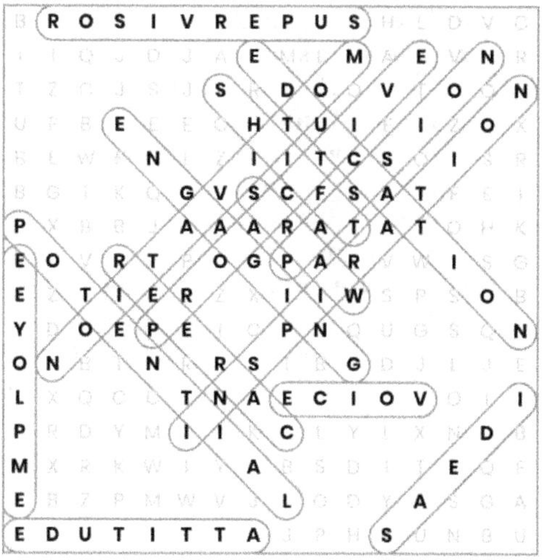

Every Second Matters - Solution

Frontline Insights and Perspectives from a 2nd Shift SPD Leader

HITSF	SHIFT	H 8, T 4
SIEVUROPSR	SUPERVISOR	U 11
MTOVOIAITN	MOTIVATION	
EEYOPMLE	EMPLOYEE	L 15, Y 5, E 19
SRWA	WARS	
EUCAIOTDN	EDUCATION	D 18, U 1, I 23
ENGGINAG	ENGAGING	E 16, G 12
PCTOVIRAE	PROACTIVE	R 9
EADSI	IDEAS	
OICEV	VOICE	
CEEARR	CAREER	
PTTOEANIL	POTENTIAL	P 24, O 10, T 7
PIOASSN	PASSION	A 17, S 21
ISPOATRNIIN	INSPIRATION	N 2, I 3, R 20
AUTTIDTE	ATTITUDE	

UNITY THROUGH LEADERSHIP

Dangers on the Orient(ation) Express - Solution

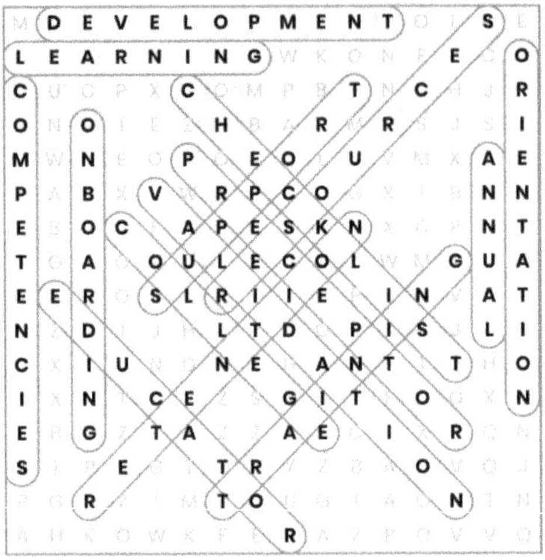

Dangers on the Orient(ation) Express - Solution

Getting On-boarding Right with Competency Based Programs

CLOEGLE	C O L L E G E	C = 1, O = 10
TNIRNIAG	T R A I N I N G	R = 11, I = 18
OINAOITERTN	O R I E N T A T I O N	N = 14, T = 15, N = 20
CIPOTENCEEMS	C O M P E T E N C I E S	O = 19, M = 3, E = 13
AUANNL	A N N U A L	A = 16, L = 5
ODABINONRG	O N B O A R D I N G	I = 12
DOEPMLNEVET	D E V E L O P M E N T	O = 2, P = 4, T = 7
EADOTCUR	E D U C A T O R	
CCLSIKHET	C H E C K L I S T	
VIOLATIDAN	V A L I D A T I O N	
POPTCERER	P R E C E P T O R	E = 6
RENTOTEIN	R E T E N T I O N	E = 8, T = 17
RCESEORUS	R E S O U R C E S	
LARNNEIG	L E A R N I N G	
SPRPUOT	S U P P O R T	

C O M P L E T E   O R I E N T A T I O N

All Together Now - Solution

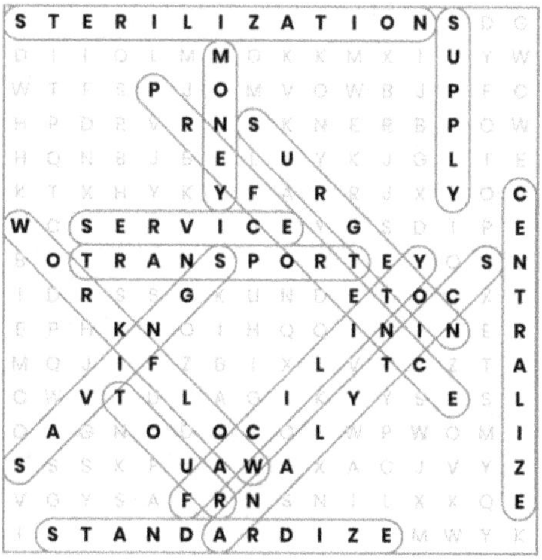

All Together Now - Solution

Sterile Processing Centralization

FIITACLY	F A C I L I T Y	
EYMON	M O N E Y	E = 10
CLENZIRTAE	C E N T R A L I Z E	C = 1, Z = 9
SDTZARNIDAE	S T A N D A R D I Z E	N = 3, D = 11
SROEUGN	S U R G E O N	R = 5, G = 22
PRFECERENE	P R E F E R E N C E	E = 2
CITNMOCAUIMON	C O M M U N I C A T I O N	O = 15, I = 20, C = 16, A = 6
SLUPPY	S U P P L Y	P = 13
SAOELITIZRITN	S T E R I L I Z A T I O N	T = 4, I = 8
TONPRRSAT	T R A N S P O R T	R = 14, N = 21, S = 19
WOFRLOKW	W O R K F L O W	L = 7
SIGNVAS	S A V I N G S	S = 18
UROT	T O U R	
AYCTIALNS	A N A L Y T I C S	
SVICERE	S E R V I C E	E = 17

C E N T R A L I Z E D P R O C E S S I N G

The Goal is Zero - Solution

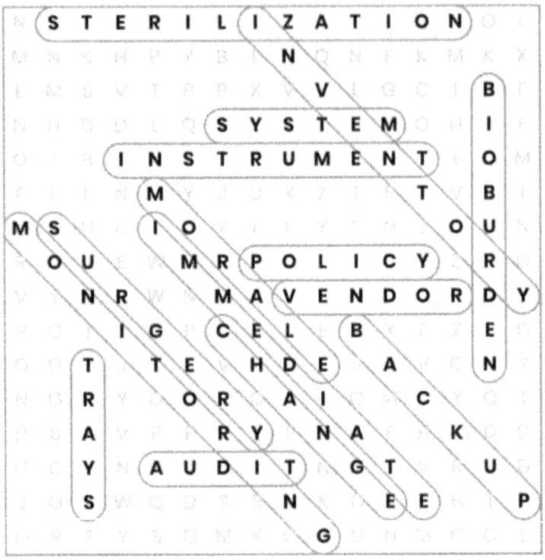

The Goal is Zero - Solution

An IUSS Success Story

BBIUEDORN	BIOBURDEN	R=13, E=14
IAEMTDIME	IMMEDIATE	A=6
VNDOER	VENDOR	
UDITA	AUDIT	U=2
CGNHAE	CHANGE	
MIOTORNNIG	MONITORING	
IVETRNNOY	INVENTORY	
PIOCLY	POLICY	O=16, I=1
SSEYTM	SYSTEM	S=15, T=18
BCUAKP	BACKUP	
IENRNMSUTT	INSTRUMENT	S=4
MRLOAE	MORALE	A=9, L=8
SIAIZTTELOIRN	STERILIZATION	S=3, T=11
RSYTA	TRAYS	S=10
SRRUGEY	SURGERY	R=17

IUSS A LAST RESORT

Reprocessing in the United Arab Emirates - Solution

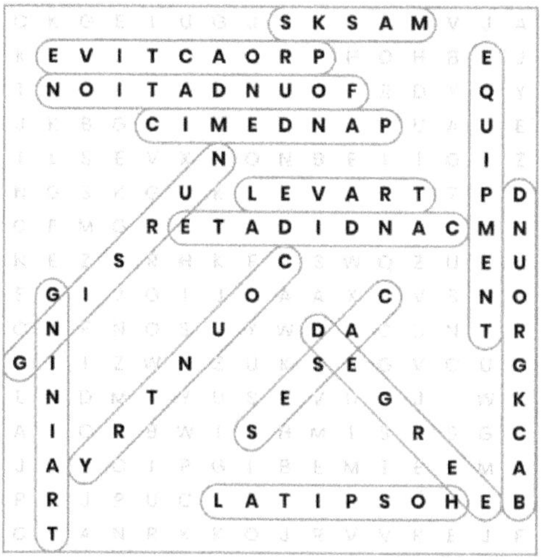

Reprocessing in the United Arab Emirates - Solution

A Story of Pandemic, Leadership & Innovation

CRTONUY	COUNTRY	C = 7
HSTIAPOL	HOSPITAL	H = 8, A = 10
DCOIEANOAMNITTN	DECONTAMINATION	D = 12, E = 4, T = 23, A = 22, M = 17
CTDAANIDE	CANDIDATE	A = 5, E = 24
NISUNRG	NURSING	R = 6
BNKACGROUD	BACKGROUND	C = 14, O = 15
DEEGRE	DEGREE	
FTOIANUODN	FOUNDATION	U = 18
TINNIARG	TRAINING	R = 1, N = 11, N = 19
PMDEAINC	PANDEMIC	E = 2
EPMQNIUET	EQUIPMENT	I = 20, M = 16
TEVRAL	TRAVEL	
KSMAS	MASKS	S = 3
SSEAC	CASES	
PIRCVOATE	PROACTIVE	C = 21

RESEARCH AND COMMUNICATE

For over 230 other CE approved podcasts, webinars, and virtual conferences visit us at beyondclean.net

Follow us on:
Linkedin:
http://www.linkedin.com/company/beyondclean

Facebook:
https://www.facebook.com/BeyondCleanPodcast/

Twitter:
https://twitter.com/beyondcleaninfo

Instagram:
https://www.instagram.com/beyondcleanpodcast/

YouTube:
https://www.youtube.com/beyondclean

CPSIA information can be obtained
at www.ICGtesting.com
Printed in the USA
BVHW091709030122
625370BV00016B/1019

9 781990 599002